Praise for *The Kitchen Commune*

"As a functional medicine expert, I understand the importance of eating healthy meals, but as a parent, getting everyone to eat well is often easier said than done. [*The Kitchen Commune*] shows us just how easy it can be to nourish everyone at your table while still providing easy customizations to account for personal taste. A game-changing book for parents and hosts alike. Say goodbye to making separate meals, and say hello to a united table!"

Dr. Will Cole, IFMCP, DNM, DC, leading functional medicine expert and bestselling author of *Ketotarian, The Inflammation Spectrum, Intuitive Fasting,* and *Gut Feelings*

"Saying Chay's recipes are incredible is quite frankly an understatement. Covering gluten-free, dairy-free, vegan, and paleo restrictions, *The Kitchen Commune* truly has something for everyone! From first-time cooks to people who have been eating with dietary restrictions most of their lives, everyone will be able to enjoy this cookbook, the recipes, and every photo in between."

Kayla Cappiello, author of *Easy Allergy-Free Cooking*

"*The Kitchen Commune* makes cooking for special diets easy by putting all the best recipes and techniques in one place and guiding [the reader] through. Chay shares her inspiring story and empowers [cooks of all levels] to cook and eat with confidence!"

Caryn Carruthers, author of *Smorgasbowl: Recipes and Techniques for Creating Satisfying Meals with Endless Variation*

"With one tempting recipe after another, *The Kitchen Commune* offers a way to satisfy diverse eating styles and health needs so loved ones can share scrumptious meals together. Chay brings food to life with such great texture, flavor, and piquancy. You'll return to the book over and over."

Kristine Kidd, former *Bon Appétit* food editor and author of *Weeknight Gluten Free*

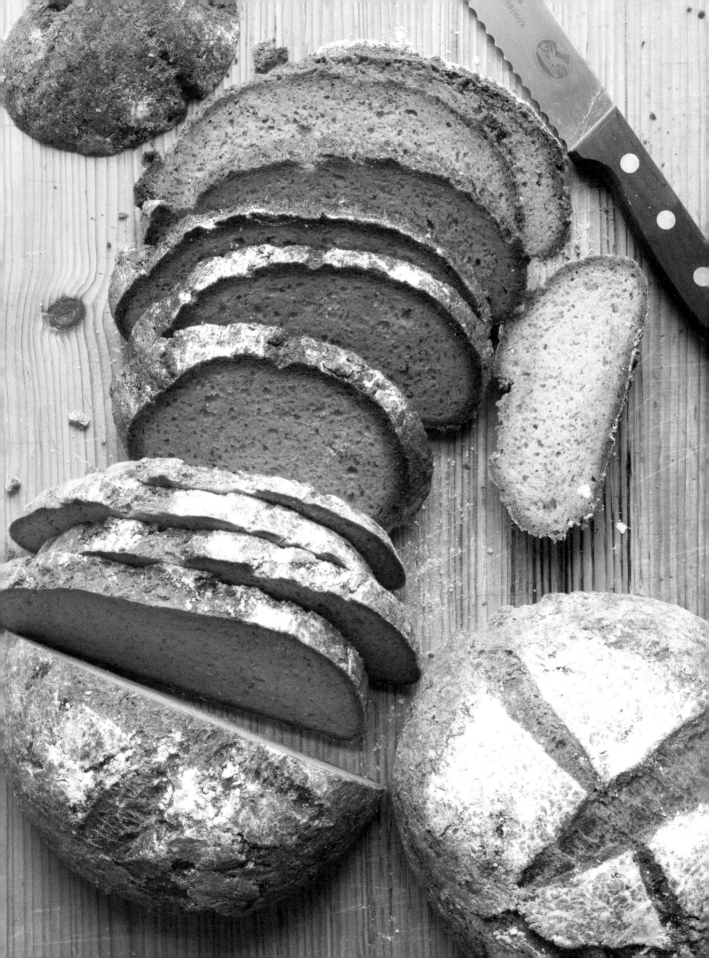

THE KITCHEN COMMUNE

MEALS TO HEAL AND NOURISH EVERYONE AT YOUR TABLE

100+ easy allergen-friendly recipes, including gluten free, paleo, vegan, and more

Chay Wike

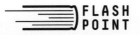

Published by Flashpoint™ Books, Seattle
www.flashpointbooks.com

Produced by Girl Friday Productions
Photography: Chay Wike
Design: Debbie Berne
Development & editorial: Leslie Jonath and Jess Thomson
Production editorial: Abi Pollokoff
Project management: Emilie Sandoz-Voyer

ISBN (hardcover): 978-1-959411-18-5
ISBN (ebook): 978-1-959411-19-2

Library of Congress Control Number: 2023903792
First edition

For Mark, Jane, and Rose
Lalu
Always and forever

Contents

ix	Introduction
xiii	The 10 Principles of *The Kitchen Commune*
xiv	Building an Alternative Pantry

Sauces + Staples

5	House Chimichurri
6	Green Onion Salsa
7	Cilantro-Mint Chutney
8	Three Dressings
10	House Pesto
11	Creamy Thai Pesto
12	Cheesy Garlic Croutons
15	Fresh Almond Ricotta Cheese
16	Fresh Almond Cream
17	Confit Three Ways
21	Chipotle Aioli
22	Smashed Cumin Guacamole
25	Caper-Currant Relish
26	Sticky Plum BBQ Sauce
28	Quick Pickles
31	Coconut Yogurt Tzatziki
32	Vanilla Berry Compote
34	Spiced Toasted Seeds
37	Toasted Plantain Crumbs
38	Bone Broth
40	Big Batch of Beans
44	Big Batch of Short-Grain Rice

Mornings

50	Super Green Veg + Fruit Shake
53	Creamy Overnight Seed Pudding
54	Grain-Free Granola
57	Fluffy Silver Dollar Pancakes
58	Wild Blueberry Muffins
61	Maple Bacon + Veg
62	Beans, Greens + Broken Eggs
65	Tinned Fish Breakfast Salad

Salads + Small Plates

70	Butter Lettuce with Fresh Herbs, Toasted Maple Sunflower Seeds + Marlit's Vinaigrette
73	Caesar Salad with Avocado, Croutons + Hemp Seeds
74	Tuscan Kale Salad with Pomegranate, Pine Nuts + Currants
77	Chicory Chop Salad
78	Heirloom Tomato Salad
81	Mandarin, Avocado + Watercress Salad
82	Curried Wild Tuna Salad

Soups + Stews

88	Bone Broth Vegetable Purée
91	Rotisserie Chicken Soup
92	Awase Dashi
95	Red Lentil Mulligatawny Soup
96	Clams with Ginger-Coconut Broth
99	White Bean + Chorizo Stew
100	Black Friday Korma

Pasta + Noodles

106	Penne alla Rosé
109	Lemon Spaghetti
110	Tagliatelle Bolognese

113 Cacio e Pepe 2.0

114 Eggplant Moussaka Bake with Fresh Almond Ricotta

117 Creamy Pad Thai Kelp Noodles

Vegetables

122 Steak Knife Roasted Vegetables

124 Crispy Brussels Sprouts with Fish Sauce Caramel

127 Pan-Sautéed Baby Turnips with Turnip Green Pesto

128 Pan-Roasted Cauliflower with Caper-Currant Relish + Yogurt-Tahini Sauce

130 Cauliflower Cannellini Bean Mash

131 Garlicky Greens with Apple Cider Vinegar

133 Roasted Honeynut Squash

134 Wild Mushrooms with Ghee, Herbs + Sherry Vinegar

137 Crispy Oven-Fried Sweet Potatoes

138 Span-ish Frittata with Spinach

Seafood

145 Citrus-Cured Lox

148 Crispy Broiled King Salmon

151 Whole Roasted Branzino

152 Seared Scallops with Garlic Ghee

155 Fried Oysters with Remoulade Sauce

156 Wild Fried Fish Tacos with Quick Pickled Slaw + Chipotle Aioli

159 Whole Garlic Prawns with Charred Lemon

160 Flounder Meunière

Poultry + Meat

166 Gochujang Wings

169 Chicken Liver Pâté

170 "Sour Cream" + Onion Chicken Thigh Schnitzel with Chip Crumbs

173 Chicken Thighs with Green Olives, Dates, Lemon + Butter Lettuce

174 Overnight Roast Chicken

177 Turkey Zucchini Patties with Coconut Yogurt Tzatziki

178 Middle Eastern Spiced Ground Bison

181 Grilled Skirt Steak with House Chimichurri

182 Slow-Roasted Ribs with Sticky Plum BBQ Sauce

185 Carnitas

186 Grass-Fed Rack of Lamb

189 Lamb Koftas

Bread, Baking + Sweets

194 Flatbreads

197 Tortillas

201 Grain-Free Vegan Boule

205 Nut + Seed Bread

209 Heirloom Tomato Galette

211 Caramel Pear Galette

215 Grain-Free Dark Chocolate Cake with Chocolate Sweet Potato Frosting

217 Carrot Birthday Cake with Cultured Buttercream + Rainbow Sprinkles

220 Shortbread Tea Biscuits

222 Date + Cacao Truffles

225 Vanilla Ice Cream

227 Resources

228 Acknowledgments

230 Index

236 About the Author

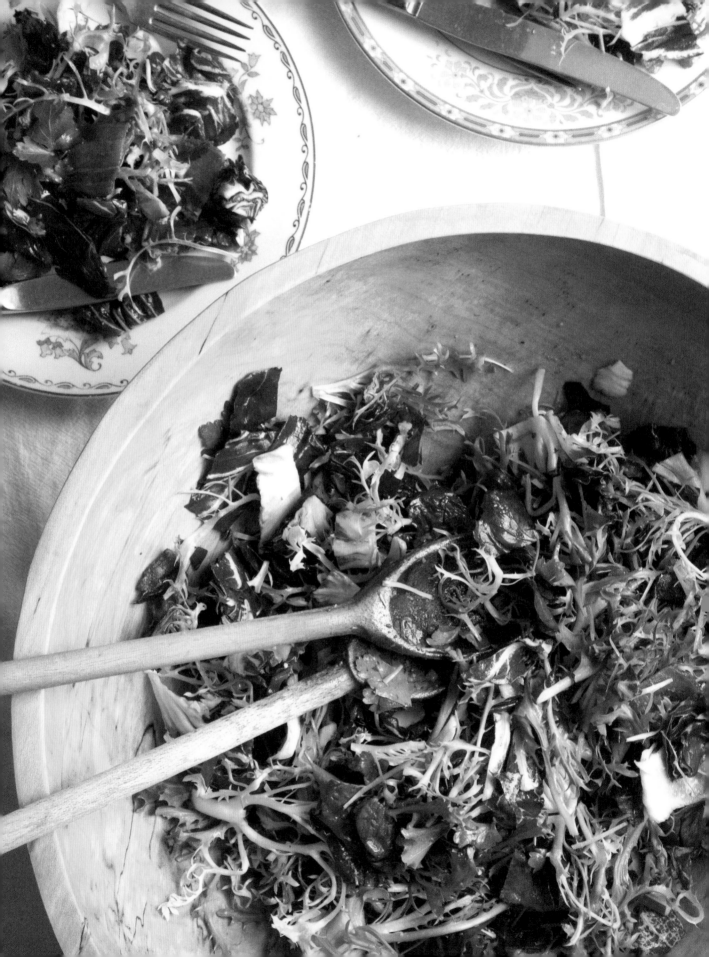

Introduction

You're a guest at a holiday meal and the host has prepared a gorgeous spread. There's a giant turkey shellacked with butter, sourdough stuffing, creamy whipped potatoes, a big salad, and the requisite pumpkin pie—the works. You don't want to draw attention to yourself, but having discovered which foods your body likes, you know you can eat only one or maybe two of the dishes laid out before you due to allergies or intolerances. You have a choice: you can nurse the salad with no dressing and submit to stares when you dig for the unbuttered part of the turkey or go for it all, knowing it may take days to recover.

Or maybe it's a weeknight, you have four kids and a partner to feed, and your stepson has a dairy allergy. Do you make him a separate meal or just give him plain pasta, again? Or perhaps it's your birthday and you decide to have a fun alfresco gathering and you know that two of your guests are vegan and one has celiac disease (i.e., can't eat gluten). Should you prepare special options for them? If so, what do those look like?

I've been there, at all those dinner tables. And I imagine you have been at similar tables, too. Every time different eating habits collide, we have questions: Do we need to sacrifice our health to be socially graceful? How high are the hoops we jump through to accommodate others? Can eating for health be desirable and delicious and enjoyable? The questions are endless, and as more of us are becoming attentive and mindful eaters, one seems loudest: Can we really eat joyfully together?

Luckily, there's a clear answer to this final question: Yes. By cooking thoughtfully, and reframing our kitchen habits around what's good for all of us rather than what's good for just one

or two people, we can keep everyone healthy without ostracizing anyone or sacrificing our own needs. We can feed the whole table. *This* is the kitchen commune.

Feeding yourself and the people you love is a powerful act. Communal dining unites us and has lasting effects on our physical and spiritual well-being. It strengthens our connections, builds trust, and releases hormones that improve digestion and mood. With a little patience and understanding, we can easily make room for each other at the table without too much trouble and get on with the pleasures and joys of eating beautiful food together.

This book will help you bridge the gaps between different health needs and eating styles one meal at a time. Having been on a health journey for 15 years and counting, I understand the courage it takes to make lasting changes to our eating habits and the challenges of sustaining them alongside family and friends. In these pages, you will learn how to simplify, unify, and streamline considerate menu planning. There's a little something in here for everyone and every occasion: I've included easy weekday breakfasts, lunches, and dinners as well as holiday entrées, desserts, and simple dishes to feed a crowd. There will also be valuable cooking techniques, tips, and health information throughout to help you grow into a more intuitive, mindful, and confident home cook. Once you understand a few basic principles (page xiii), you'll learn that you can combine dishes and ingredients to create a well-rounded meal that everyone in your own kitchen commune can enjoy.

XO

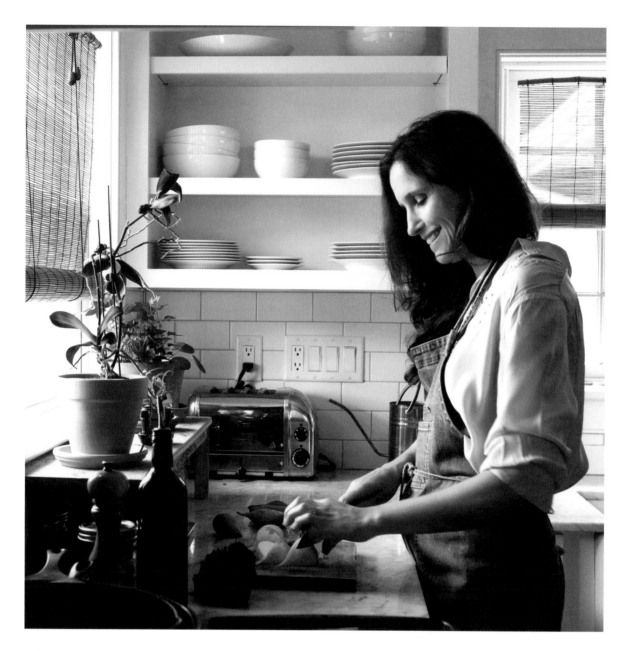

About Me

I come from a family of self-taught home cooks and homemakers. I've been cooking since I was a teenager. As with some of us, my best memories are of my grandmothers in their kitchens. Making meals and *serving* them to the people I love, in my home, is in my blood and brings me

a deep sense of purpose. I take enormous pride in creating a sanctuary that provides a place to restore and nourish my family. I grew up in New York City, but my parents and grandparents are from Cape Town, South Africa. I had the privilege of traveling overseas during the holidays and being exposed to all kinds of cultures and eating styles from an early age. My parents are divorced, so growing up I spent alternating weeks with each parent, living between their two apartments. My mother cooked homemade meals every day and set the table for breakfast and dinner. From her, I learned that eating begins long before your food arrives and that setting a table has a way of stopping time and shifting gears. While I was in my tiny bedroom doing homework, I could smell her chicken roasting or her salmon steaks crisping in the broiler. She kept a lovely home and made real suppers, always served with a fresh salad tossed in homemade vinaigrette. My father, on the other hand, worked very late and long hours, so I did most of the cooking at his place. He also took me out to eat Indian, Japanese, Italian, Middle Eastern, and Mexican food, constantly broadening my culinary horizons.

Today, I live in the Pennsylvania countryside with my husband and our two teenage daughters. My life changed dramatically after the birth of our second child, in 2006, when my health started to decline. After several years of testing, I was finally diagnosed with multiple autoimmune conditions, digestive issues, and (eventually) Lyme disease. Following a string of confusing doctor visits and failed medication attempts, I decided to take matters into my own hands and reclaim my health naturally by changing my eating habits.

Before I made the connection between my health and my food, I was eating everything without any hesitation. I *love* to eat. However, once I realized that the food I was eating was having a major impact on my health, it became impossible to ignore that I needed to make a change. I saw altering my diet as my path to healing. In 2009, I attended a traditional cooking school in Los Angeles to take my home-cooking skills to the next level so I could apply them to cooking with alternative ingredients. I have since

mostly recovered, using the undeniable power of functional nutrition and lifestyle medicine. I went on to launch a food-focused wellness blog called *The Kitchen Commune* in 2018, sharing some of the recipes I've developed for myself and others along the way. Shortly after that, in 2020, I became a certified integrative health coach and began focusing on helping others heal, too.

Over the course of my health journey, I have committed to several diets and practices, one after the next, in search of recovery. I've experimented with the blood type diet, the bean protocol, the autoimmune protocol, the Ayurvedic diet, the macrobiotic diet, and Ohsawa Diet #7. I've tried vegan, paleo, keto, and pescatarian diets. I've fasted, I've sweat, I've journeyed, I've retreated, I've mantra'd, I've meditated. I've seen intuitives, astrologers, and shamans. I've done acupuncture, colonics, cupping, intravenous light therapy, and intravenous ozone therapy, and traveled far and wide to see special people who do special things that nobody knows about. I've done all of this because, at points along the way, I've had flare-ups that have landed me in the hospital and I've faced my mortality. I would go to the end of the earth and back to heal my precious body, because I understand intimately that I get only one in this life. None of those special diets or therapies was a magic bullet, but each of them gave me valuable information and pieces of the puzzle I needed to solve, and over the years I have cobbled together a personal health plan unique to my needs. The recipes in this book reflect everything I've learned along the way, but I'm certain there's something in here for you, too. Whether you are curious about health or a seasoned self-healer, or simply want to make beautiful meals that accommodate a wide variety of diets, I'm confident you can find recipes for you and your loved ones herein.

What Is and Isn't Here

I've spent the last 15 years developing recipes and strategies in the kitchen that take my health needs and my family's cravings into consideration. On this health journey, I've found a way to rework many of our favorite foods so that they don't cause real trouble in my body. I still eat pasta and tacos and cake, because I have learned to make them my way. What you'll find in these pages is the result of years of fine-tuning the art of eating together—family-friendly recipes and inspiration that are free of gluten and refined sugar yet full of flavor, texture, and richness. There will be no sense of lacking or restriction, but instead an emphasis on whole foods and classics updated with ingredients that more people can eat and the connective magic of sauce. (See Sauce It on page xiii.)

All the recipes in this book are gluten-free and virtually dairy-free (see Ghee on page xiv), but they are much more than that. They are designed to be nutrient-dense as well, because chances are if you are choosing to eat this way (or someone you know is), you are probably trying to rebalance your body in some way, or to simply heal. Foods that tend to cause the least amount of inflammation or flare-ups include fruits, vegetables, healthy fats, and clean animal and fish proteins.

Many of the recipes intentionally avoid some foods that can be difficult to digest or absorb for some people. For example, while I occasionally include rice, beans, soy, and eggs, the majority of the recipes in the book are free of them.

Nightshades are a family of plants that include some common edible fruits and vegetables which can be problematic for some people, too. These include tomatoes, white potatoes, bell peppers, chilies, and eggplant, and chili-based spices like red pepper flakes, paprika, and cayenne. I do not tolerate nightshades all that well but have found that I can have them in small amounts occasionally. There are only a few recipes that feature nightshades in the book, but otherwise you should be able to easily omit them from recipes if necessary.

My wish for you, in cooking from these pages, is to celebrate inclusive eating and discover that it's much easier than you imagined. Once you realize that there is plenty of common ground from which you can build delicious meals regardless of different eating styles, you will be well on your way to thoughtful cooking for your own kitchen commune.

The 10 Principles of *The Kitchen Commune*

1   Sauce It

Sauce is the universal connector at the table. Making sauces ahead of time enriches meals because you can serve them with everything, and the experience brings people together at the table.

2   Cook for the Week

Make a big pot of stew or rice, or a double batch of meatballs over the weekend to have on hand all week long. (See Cooking for Your Future Self on page 121.)

3   Think in Threes

If possible, try to have three simple dishes rather than one big dish. For example, a salad, a pot of beans, and a roast chicken. This allows people to customize their plates.

4   Find Your Go-To Dishes

Master a few recipes that accommodate any dietary considerations in your circle of friends and family and that cover all the bases for easy family-style dining.

5   Source the Best

Always try to use very good ingredients: find quality organic fruits and vegetables, wild fish, and pastured poultry and meat. (See Making Choices at the Meat Counter on page 165.)

6   Go Alternative

Become familiar with starch alternatives like gluten-free whole grains, beans, pulses, and root vegetables, which are all filling and provide a satisfying substitute for gluten. They also appeal to mostly everyone. Make sure you use the best gluten-free pasta you can find and learn how to cook it properly, so any skeptics can discover it stands up well to their expectations.

7   Bring on the Healthy Fats

Healthy fats are good for all; they help us absorb vital nutrients, give us energy, and provide satiety. Keep the olive oil, olives, ghee, coconut oil, avocados, nuts, and seeds flowing.

8   Deconstruct Dishes

Serve meals with gluten, dairy, sauces, or any known allergens on the side so loved ones can mix and match based on dietary choices. Allow people to customize their plates without a spotlight.

9   Set the Table

Whether it's with flowers or simple paper plates, setting the table invites us to celebrate the ritual of sharing a meal every day.

10   Be Kind and Curious

Embracing the dietary diversity we find at every table means not judging yourself or others for the choices we all make. Being kind to yourself also means staying curious about food. Finding healthier, more mindful eating habits doesn't mean shutting out new foods.

Building an Alternative Pantry

Becoming familiar with alternative ingredients and keeping a well-stocked pantry will help you maintain and sustain your health efforts and get meals on the table more easily. Here are some of my favorite substitute ingredients and staple pantry items that I use most frequently. While they're more expensive, I try to invest in as many organic products as I can find and afford. I consider this to be part of my out-of-pocket health expenses.

Healthy Fats + Nut Butters + Oils

Ghee
Ghee is a type of clarified butter. Clarified butter is butter that has been melted and cooked to separate and remove the milk solids from the butter fat. For ghee, the milk solids are left in the melted butter longer to caramelize before they are removed, creating a nutty flavor profile. It is not 100 percent dairy-free, but it has only trace amounts of dairy that can often be tolerated by individuals with dairy sensitivities. I use it instead of regular butter for sautéing, making baked goods, and enriching sauces, and to smear over toast. It does not need to be refrigerated because most of the dairy has been removed. I store mine in the pantry.

Extra-Virgin Olive Oil
I use extra-virgin olive oil the most in my cooking. Olive oil is made from pressed or crushed whole fresh olives. There are an overwhelming number of varietals and types of oil to choose from. My favorites are from Greece and Spain. Extra-virgin olive oil is made from the first cold pressing of the fruit, which means it is unrefined, contains the most nutrients, and is pricier than other grades of oil. I like olive oil that has a peppery aftertaste with some kick to it. There are some olive varietals that can withstand higher cooking temperatures, but in general it's better not to use this oil to fry with. I use it for sautéing, roasting chicken, making salad dressings or sauces, and for finishing.

Avocado Oil
Avocado oil is extracted from the pulp of avocados. It has a neutral flavor profile and a high smoke point, making it an ideal frying oil. I like to use it in baked goods as well.

Coconut Oil
Coconut oil comes from the kernel of mature coconut palm fruit. It is solid and stored at room temperature. It can be easily melted and is a great vegan substitute for baking and cooking when you need to replace butter or ghee.

Coconut Butter
This is made from puréed mature coconut meat that is ground into a thick paste. It can become solid at room temperature and sometimes needs to be gently heated up to become creamy.

Almond Butter
Almond butter is a thick paste of ground almonds that can be smooth or crunchy. I look for brands that don't have any added oils or sugar. Some grocery stores have self-serve fresh-nut-grinding machines that make instant nut butters on the spot.

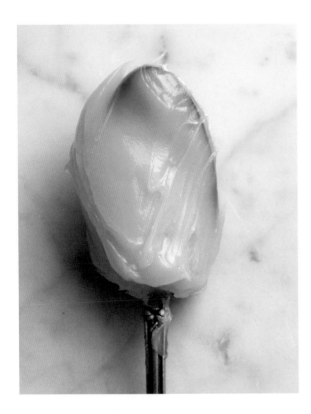

Grain-Free Flours + Binders

Superfine Almond Flour
This is different from almond meal in that it is made from skinless blanched almonds, which makes it more easily digestible for some people. I use this a lot for baking. It adds structure and healthy fats to baked goods.

Cassava Flour
Cassava, also known as yuca, is a starchy vegetable in the tuber family. It is dried and ground into a flour that can be used in a wide variety of baked goods. Not all cassava flour is alike, as some can produce undesirable results. I like Otto's and Bob's Red Mill brands.

Coconut Flour
This is made from dried ground coconut meat. I use it in baking sometimes to add structure to cakes and muffins.

Tapioca Flour
This is a starch extracted from the cassava root. It helps add fluffiness to baked goods and crunchiness to crusts.

Arrowroot Flour
This starchy powder is extracted from the root of a tropical plant called *Maranta arundinacea*. It can be used as a thickening agent and to lighten the texture of baked goods. It can also be used as a binder.

Cacao Powder
Not to be confused with cocoa powder, cacao powder is minimally processed and contains higher levels of antioxidants. I use this to add deep chocolatiness to cakes and truffles.

Ground Flaxseed or Flaxseed Meal
Flaxseed is a plant-based food that is high in fiber and omega-3 fatty acids. I use it in baked goods sometimes as an egg replacer or binder, and to add structure. It also helps to thicken smoothies and boost nutrition.

Psyllium Husk
Psyllium husk is a form of fiber made from the outer coating of seeds that come from the *Plantago ovata* plant. It is mostly a soluble fiber, and I use it in baked goods as a binder. It comes both in whole husk form and as a powder, so pay attention to the packaging when you purchase it.

Dairy Alternatives

Almond Milk
This is the milk I use the most and find it works well in all baked goods and batters. I look for brands that have two ingredients: almonds and water. There are many brands that contain gums, starches, industrial seed oils, and other things that don't need to be in nut milk.

Almond Cream

This is a nondairy almond-based cream that is similar to half-and-half in consistency. I make mine from scratch (page 16) and use it in tea, coffee, and sauces. It is rich and concentrated. A little goes a long way. The flavor is neutral, and I love how it enriches everything I add it to.

Canned Full-Fat Coconut Milk or Cream

Coconut milk and cream both come from coconut, but the cream has a much higher fat content. I make sure to seek out brands that are 100 percent pure and free of gums and thickeners. I use this in baked goods, sauces, and curries, and to make vegan ice cream.

Coconut Yogurt

Coconut yogurt is a vegan yogurt made from coconut milk. I use this in baked goods, as a base for sauces, and as a substitute for mayonnaise. I make sure to find brands that do not use any gums or fillers. You can also strain it to make a thick Greek-style yogurt.

Minimally Processed Natural Sweeteners

Maple Syrup

Maple syrup is vegan and made from the sap of maple trees. It used to be available in two different grades, but this system was officially changed in 2015. Today, there are still two different kinds of maple syrup, but they are both classified as Grade A. One is dark and the other very dark. The first one is produced at the beginning of the season and is lighter in color and slightly sweeter. The second, darker syrup is produced later in the season and is thicker and richer in flavor. I use the latter in baking and sauces because it blends easily and has a caramel-like flavor profile.

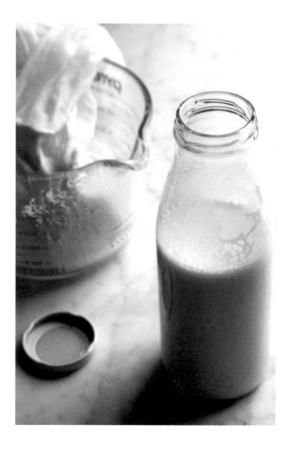

Honey

Honey is not considered to be vegan, because it is made by bees. Raw honey is preferable to pasteurized because it contains more antioxidants. It's also a good idea to try to source it locally if possible because it contains local pollen that will help strengthen your immune system and might help with allergies. I like to smear it on toast or drizzle it over yogurt.

Coconut Sugar

Coconut sugar is a palm sugar made from coconut palm sap; it's less processed than regular table sugar. I like to use it in baking and sauces.

Dates

Dates are a sweet stone fruit from date palm trees that are native to the Middle East. I particularly like Medjool dates from Morocco because

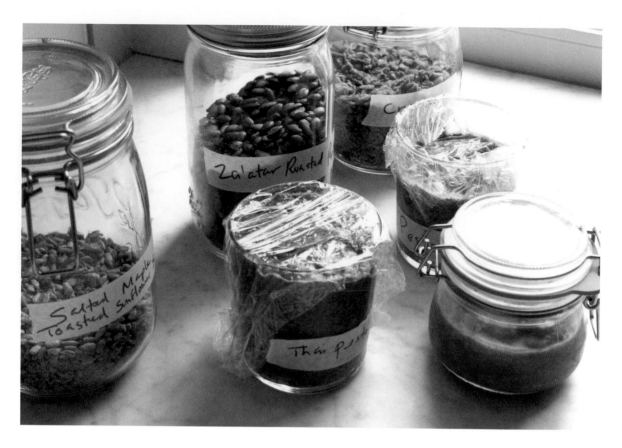

they are plump. They can be a lovely substitute for sugar and lend themselves very well to baking and cooking. I like to blend them whole into dough for chocolate truffles and roast them alongside chicken.

Seasoning + Spices

Kosher Sea Salt
Kosher sea salt typically has a larger flake size, making it easier to grab when seasoning food. Every recipe in this book uses kosher sea salt and is measured accordingly.

Freshly Ground Black Pepper
I use pepper sparingly. At one point I had mold toxicity in my body and my doctor advised me to limit pre-ground pepper because it tends to have mold in it. Freshly ground black pepper can help to reduce mold exposure.

Alcohol-Free Vanilla Extract
I prefer to use alcohol-free vanilla extract (except in my vanilla ice-cream recipe, where alcohol is needed to help prevent ice crystals) because it is thick and syrupy and lends itself really well to baking. I also use it as a sugar-free sweetener for my tea.

Nutritional Yeast
This is a deactivated form of yeast used in cooking that brings a savory, cheesy flavor to baked goods and sauces, and is totally vegan. I prefer natural non-fortified nutritional yeast, as it is already full of B vitamins, protein, and fiber.

Bottles + Tins + Jars

Coconut Aminos
This is a soy-free liquid condiment made from the fermented sap of a coconut palm tree and sea salt. I use it to season stir-fries and sauces and as an alternative to soy sauce for dipping sushi.

Tamari
This is a Japanese gluten-free soy sauce made from fermented soybeans. I use it sparingly to season stir-fries and sauces.

Fish Sauce
This is a complex liquid condiment made from salt-packed fermented fish. It has a funky, salty flavor profile and adds depth and umami to sauces, marinades, and stir-fries.

Vinegar
Vinegar is an acidic and sour condiment usually made by fermenting sweet substances like fruit or wine. I love apple cider vinegar for its cooked-fruit flavor profile; balsamic vinegar has notes of molasses and prune; champagne vinegar is light and fruity; sherry vinegar has notes of tawny port; and rice vinegar is delicately sweet compared to other vinegars. I suggest you start collecting them and play around. I use them to balance out sauces and salad dressings and to pickle vegetables.

Wild Tuna Fish
This is preserved wild tuna fish that comes in a glass jar and is found in most large grocery stores and many specialty markets. I prefer olive oil–packed fish because I love the extra fat. Tuna is a deep-sea fish that is higher in mercury compared to most other fish, so it should be eaten in moderation. I love to make my Curried Wild Tuna Salad (page 82) with it, or sometimes just have it straight from the jar over mixed greens.

Tinned Fish
This is preserved olive oil–packed seafood that comes in a tin and includes sardines, anchovies, trout, mackerel, mussels, salmon, cockles, octopus, and squid. These are found in most large grocery stores and specialty markets. I love to eat tinned fish for a quick savory breakfast and also find them great for travel, especially if you have dietary considerations. They also make fun gifts as they can come in cool packaging.

Olives
Olives are very high in vitamin E and other powerful antioxidants. They are a wonderful source of healthy fats. There are so many varietals to choose from. My favorites are Castelvetrano and Botija. I eat them as snacks, put them in salads and on charcuterie boards, and roast them with chicken or fish.

Capers
Capers are edible flower buds that grow on a perennial plant called *Capparis spinosa*. They have a briny lemony and tart flavor profile. They usually come in glass jars. I chop them up and add them to sauces and also sauté them with ghee and seafood.

Tomato Paste
This is a concentrated paste made of tomatoes that have been cooked and reduced for several hours. The skin and seeds have been strained out as well. I use this sparingly to add depth and umami to sauces, stews, soups, and ground meat.

Country-Style Dijon Mustard
This version of Dijon mustard is coarsely ground and has a thicker texture than regular Dijon mustard. I find it to be an ideal emulsifier for making salad dressing.

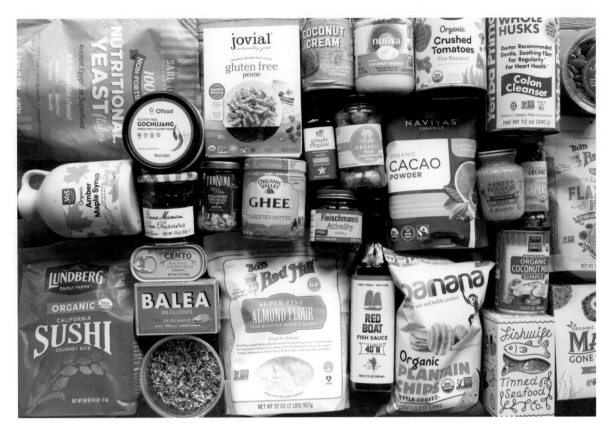

Canned Beans

These are very convenient and great to have on hand for nutritious impromptu meal assembly. I prefer unsalted beans and make sure to rinse them well before cooking.

Dry Goods

Short-Grain Rice

Short-grain rice contains more starch than long-grain. The grains are plump and stickier than other kinds of rice. I prefer the texture of this kind of rice and serve it plain alongside meat, fish, chicken, and vegetables with a rich sauce.

Gluten-Free Pasta

Gluten-free pasta is made without wheat and instead from either rice, corn, quinoa, lentils, or beans, or a combination of a few things. There are some really special brands that make

spectacular products. My favorite is Jovial. Their noodles are made in Italy using traditional production methods.

Dried Beans

Beans are a legume high in fiber, folate, potassium, iron, and magnesium. With well over 400 types of varietals, they are easily found in most grocery stores. Some of my favorites include cannellini, pinto, black, and kidney. I like to make a big pot of beans full of herbs, broth, and aromatics to have in the fridge on a regular basis.

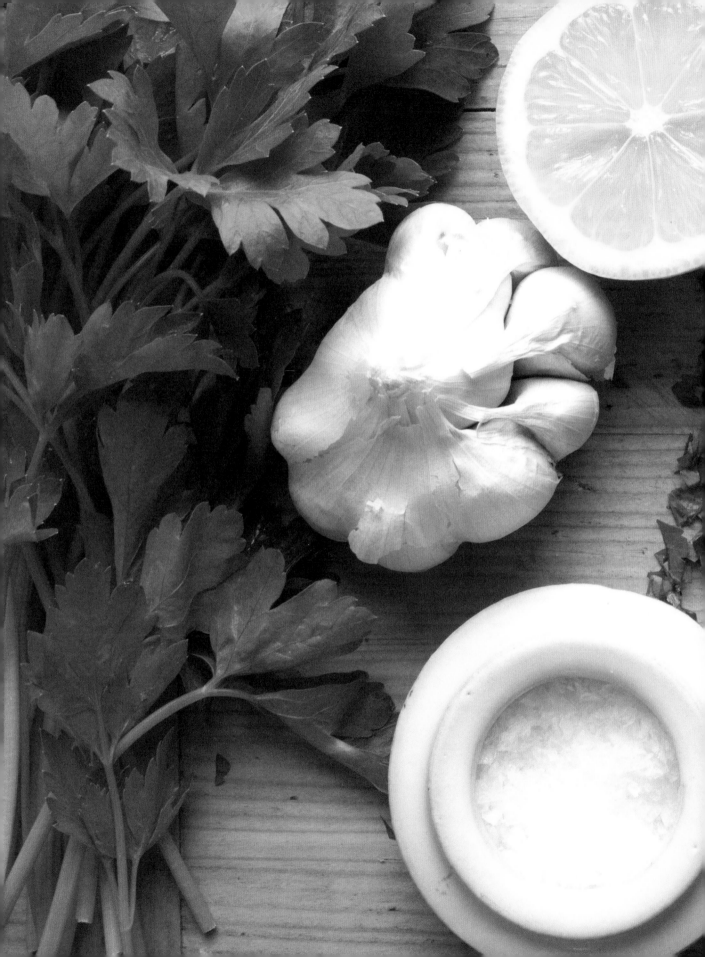

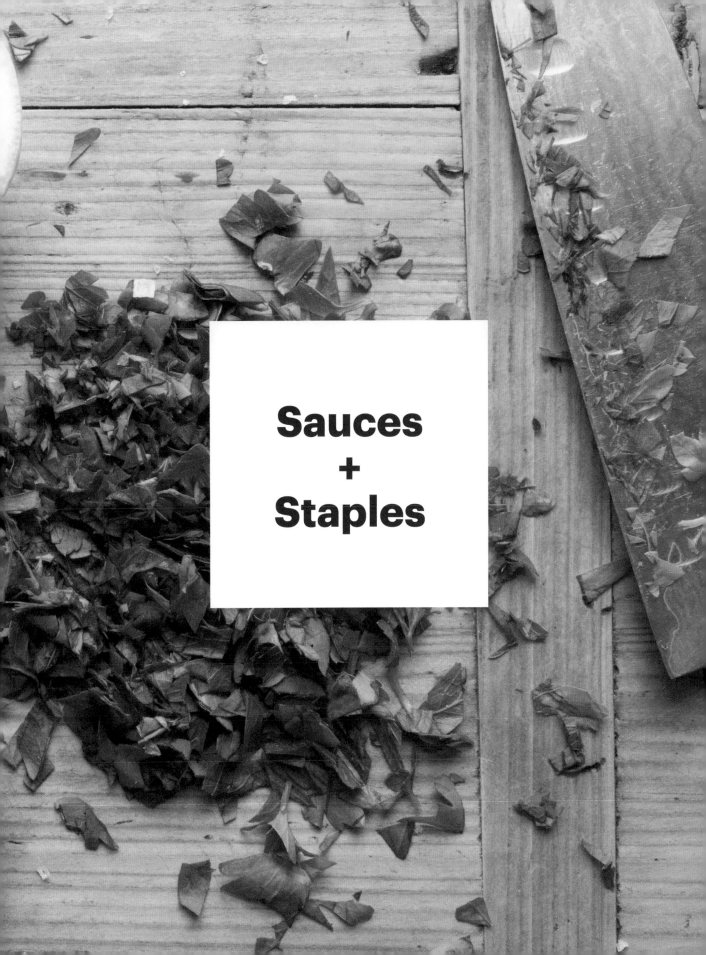

Sauces
+
Staples

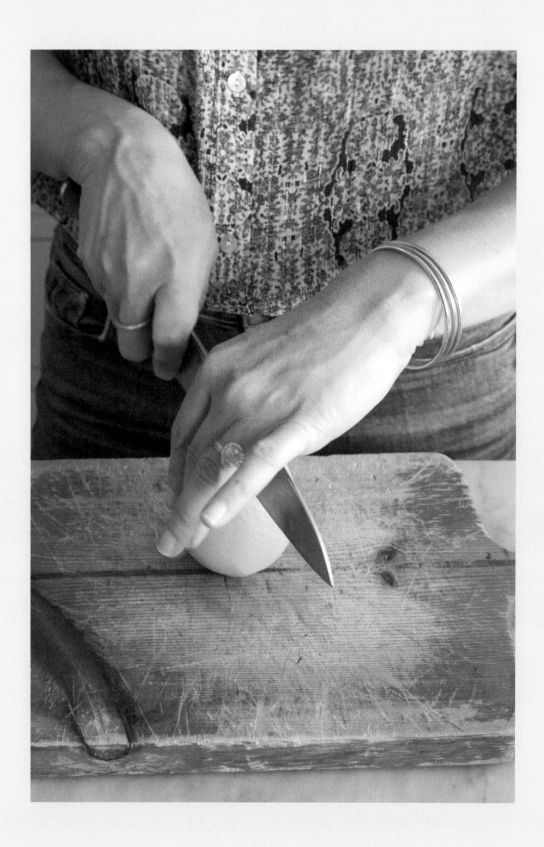

Becoming an Intuitive Cook

senses + repetition + time = intuitive cooking

What does *intuitive cooking* mean? For me, it's all about trusting your instincts without needing to rely on a recipe. Simply put, intuition is a gut feeling. Intuitive cooking means following that feeling when it comes to preparing your food and knowing when it's ready for the table. It's adding more salt or more lemon, or letting a protein cook just a little bit longer, or learning how large you like to cut your vegetables. The process comes more easily for some of us than for others, but we all have an innate guiding system, and with practice anyone can learn to use it more.

Writing this book was challenging because, truthfully, unless I'm baking, I don't use recipes! I appreciate and understand the value of having a recipe and why we absolutely need them, but I've learned to cook over time through the use of my senses and repetition. I've developed the ability to make smarter decisions while cooking that have become automatic and produce successful outcomes more regularly. I've gotten to know my food intimately. I know how it behaves, and how it should look, smell, sound, feel, and taste while I'm cooking. If you pay attention and use *all* your senses, eventually your intuition will develop, and you can relax into your cooking.

The best way to do this is to practice, and making sauce is a great place to start. For one thing, it's a very forgiving process. You can taste and adjust ingredients easily as you go until the flavors are well balanced to your liking. Pick a sauce in this next chapter like the House Pesto (page 10) and make it 10 times. Yes, 10 TIMES. Eventually you will get a *feel* for it and discover that you don't need the recipe anymore. It's not just memorization; you're developing your senses. Over time your repertoire will naturally expand as you make things multiple times, and you'll have your own little world going on in your kitchen.

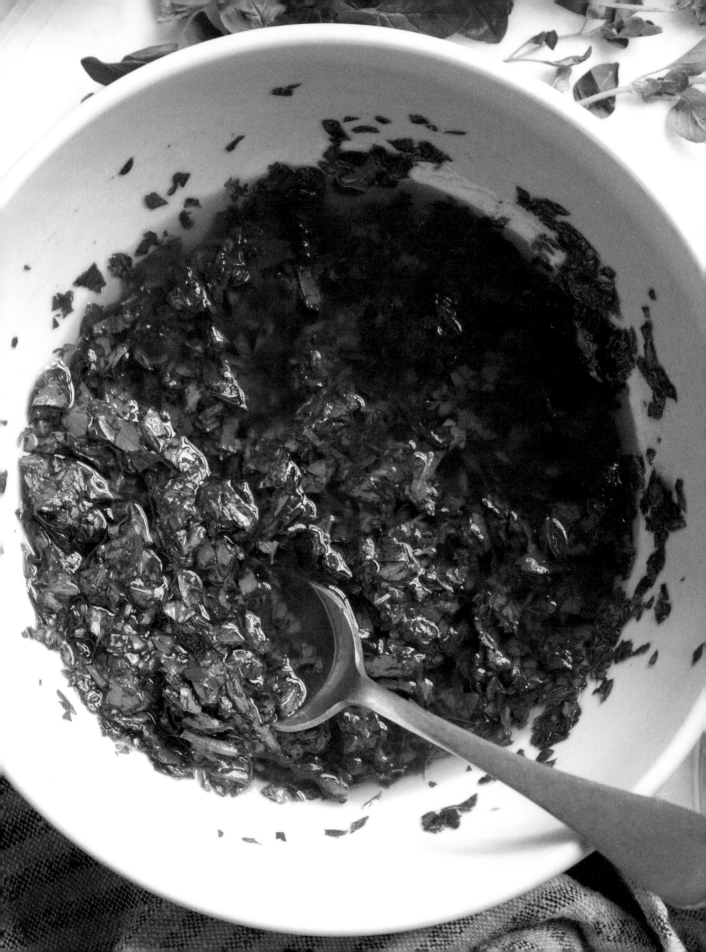

House Chimichurri

This might be the number one sauce in our home. Chimichurri is an herby, punchy, oil-based condiment that originates from Argentina and Uruguay and is typically served alongside grilled meats. There are so many variations out there, but traditionally it's a looser sauce, made of parsley, oregano, garlic, chilies, vinegar, olive oil, and salt. I've left out the nightshades here and added a dash of maple syrup and some fresh lemon to balance it out and build in some more flavor. I think my kids would be happy to put a straw into the bowl and drink it straight up! We serve this with almost everything from steak, chicken, fish, and eggs to veggies, rice, beans, and bread. I've also used it as a salad dressing. Perhaps it's the Swiss Army knife of sauces? I hope you pass the bowl around and lick your plate.

In a medium bowl, combine the parsley, garlic, oregano, lemon zest and juice, vinegar, maple syrup, and salt and stir. Slowly drizzle in the olive oil and mix the ingredients with a fork.

Adjust with vinegar, maple syrup, and salt to your liking. Use immediately, or transfer to an airtight container and refrigerate for up to a week.

Makes about 2 cups

1 cup finely chopped Italian parsley (from 1 large bunch, large stems removed)

1 large clove garlic, finely chopped or grated

1 tablespoon fresh oregano, finely chopped

Zest and juice of half a lemon

2 tablespoons red wine vinegar, plus more as needed

2 teaspoons maple syrup, plus more as needed

½ teaspoon kosher sea salt, plus more as needed

¾ cup extra-virgin olive oil

Tip
There is something special about making this sauce by hand. If you are tempted to use the food processor for the entire recipe, I encourage you to at least make it by hand once and compare the difference. The machine aerates the sauce and makes it foamy, while mixing by hand keeps it silky and luscious. Doesn't that sound better?

Green Onion Salsa

This is my play on an Italian *salsa verde*. I LOVE a bright green sauce that's packed with herbs, and the green onions here are more mellow than white or red onions, allowing this sauce to accompany rather than overpower a main dish. A hit of sweet orange juice balances out all the salty, zesty, briny flavors. The anchovy paste adds a depth of flavor without any fishiness. Serve this alongside seafood or sliced steak or spooned over rice.

In a large mortar and pestle (or in the bowl of a food processor), combine the parsley, green onion, garlic, capers, mustard, anchovy paste, salt, and lemon zest and juice, and pound or pulse until finely chopped. Transfer the mixture to a bowl and stir in the olive oil until well combined. Add the fresh orange juice and stir again.

Taste and adjust flavors if necessary.

Serve immediately, or transfer to an airtight container and store in the fridge for up to a week.

Makes about 1½ cups

½ cup roughly chopped flat-leaf parsley

½ cup roughly chopped green onion

1 small clove garlic, grated

1 tablespoon capers, roughly chopped

1 teaspoon country-style Dijon mustard

1 teaspoon anchovy paste

½ teaspoon kosher sea salt

Zest and juice of 1 small lemon

¾ cup extra-virgin olive oil

2 tablespoons freshly squeezed orange juice (from 1 medium orange)

Cilantro-Mint Chutney

One of my favorite things about Indian food is the condiment situation. I love the tray of tamarind sauce, minced onions, and cilantro-mint chutney usually served with *papadam* at Indian restaurants. This sauce is a beautifully fragrant, cool, and tangy green chutney with fresh herbs and creamy yogurt. It can be served with curry, as a lovely dipping sauce for fries and vegetables, or alongside Grass-Fed Rack of Lamb (page 186).

Place all the ingredients in an upright blender and mix until creamy and flecked with herbs, about 30 seconds. (You may need to use a spatula to push the herbs down to get the blender going as you begin.) Use immediately, or store in an airtight container in the fridge for up to a week.

Makes about 1 cup

1 cup unsweetened, plain Greek-style coconut yogurt (such as Cocojune Pure Coconut)

1 cup packed cilantro (leaves and tender stems)

½ cup packed mint leaves

1 (1-inch) piece ginger, peeled and roughly chopped

2 cloves garlic, roughly chopped

½ teaspoon kosher sea salt

1 tablespoon freshly squeezed lemon juice

1 teaspoon maple syrup

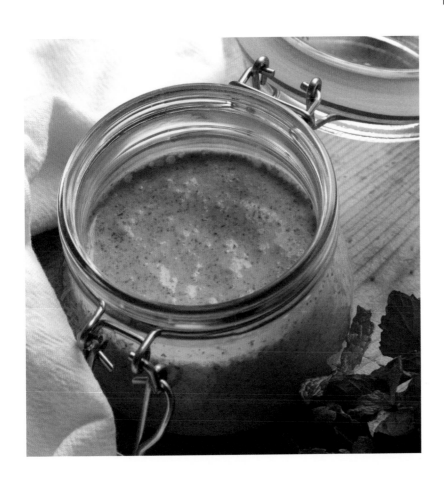

Three Dressings

In my humble opinion, there are three important things you need to know how to make when you grow up and leave home to go out into the world: roast chicken, salad, and salad dressing. Whether you eat roast chicken or not, it will come in handy and feed a crowd. A good salad requires no cooking and very little equipment. And if you can make a great salad dressing, then you can combine all three and throw a fantastic dinner party and impress your friends! Here are the three dressings I rely on most in my kitchen.

Marlit's Vinaigrette

My maternal grandmother, Marlit, escaped the Holocaust as a child and ended up in Southern France, and then eventually Paris, where she lived for many years and fell in love with the culture and cuisine before meeting my grandfather and moving with him back to South Africa in the 1950s. She was famous in our family for her salad and dressing, which I've come to understand is a classic French vinaigrette. She used regular sugar in her original recipe, but I've swapped it for maple syrup here. You could also use honey or brown sugar, if you prefer.

In a medium bowl, use a small spoon to mix the mustard, vinegar, garlic, lemon juice, maple syrup, salt, and pepper. Add 2 tablespoons of the oil and vigorously stir with a spoon until the oil incorporates into the dressing. When it no longer separates, add another 2 tablespoons of the oil and repeat. Continue adding the oil in small increments, stirring vigorously in between batches, until all the oil has been emulsified.

The dressing should be thick and well combined. Spoon over your salad immediately, or transfer the dressing to an airtight container and store it in the fridge for up to a week.

Makes about ¾ cup

1 tablespoon country-style Dijon mustard

1 tablespoon apple cider vinegar

1 large clove garlic, grated

1 teaspoon freshly squeezed lemon juice

1 teaspoon maple syrup

⅛ teaspoon kosher sea salt

Freshly ground black pepper

½ cup extra-virgin olive oil

Swap It
Feel free to use any vinegar you like and add a few tablespoons of finely chopped shallots, too.

Whole-Lemon Anchovy Dressing

This is a magically complex, lush, and lemony dressing that uses the whole lemon—peel, pith, and all—which helps create a creaminess without using any dairy. It whips up easily in a blender and can be used in an array of salads (see Chicory Chop Salad on page 77 and Heirloom Tomato Salad on page 78), where it adds deep flavor without any fishiness. You can also blend a few spoonfuls into a batch of hummus to add depth, smear some on a chicken sandwich, or brush over fish on the grill. You can halve the batch, if you want, but I find having this dressing on hand is a really helpful backup for quick meal assembly.

In an upright blender, combine all the ingredients and process for about 30 seconds, until smooth and creamy. Use immediately, or transfer to an airtight container and store in the fridge for up to a week. Bring to room temperature before serving.

Makes 2 generous cups

1 cup extra-virgin olive oil

½ cup water

1 medium whole lemon (about 5 ounces), washed clean, diced, seeds removed

1 (2-ounce) tin anchovies, drained

4 large cloves raw garlic, chopped

1 heaping tablespoon country-style Dijon mustard

Lots of freshly ground black pepper

Swap It
Substitute 7 cloves of garlic confit for the raw garlic if you have some lying around.

Caesar Dressing

I'm team anchovy all the way when it comes to Caesar dressing. It really doesn't make it fishy; it just adds lots of salty and delicious umami. Cheesy nutritional yeast is the other key ingredient here that makes this version virtually indistinguishable from the classic. It is loaded with tons of flavor and has a nice peppery kick.

Place all the ingredients in an upright blender with ½ cup of the olive oil. Blend on low to break down the lemon, garlic, and anchovies until a thick paste forms, about 10 seconds. Add the remaining olive oil and blend again until the dressing is thick and creamy, about another 10 seconds.

Taste and add more pepper if necessary. Use immediately, or transfer to an airtight container and store in the fridge for up to a week. Bring to room temperature before serving.

Makes about 2 cups

1 medium whole lemon (about 5 ounces), washed clean, diced, seeds removed

4 large cloves raw garlic, chopped

1 (2-ounce) tin anchovies, drained

1 heaping tablespoon country-style Dijon mustard

2 teaspoons Worcestershire sauce

3 tablespoons nutritional yeast

Lots of freshly ground pepper

1 cup extra-virgin olive oil, divided

House Pesto

Pesto is one of my favorite sauces because it's rich with flavor and so easy to customize to whatever your dietary needs may be. This is a very forgiving recipe that allows you to play around with ingredients or keep things very simple. Either way, you will end up with a versatile, luscious, fresh basil-based sauce that is ideal for tossing with pasta or spooning over vegetables, grains, toast, or proteins. Sometimes I even use it as salad dressing. My version is somewhat classic and uses warm toasted pine nuts for their sweet and soft nutty flavor. I don't eat dairy, so I use cheesy and tangy nutritional yeast instead of Parmesan. It's truly a perfect substitute.

Place the nuts, garlic, and salt in the bowl of a food processor and pulse a few times, until the mixture resembles wet coarse crumbs.

Scrape down the sides of the bowl with a rubber spatula, and add the rest of the ingredients. Pulse a few more times, until a thick sauce has formed.

Use immediately, or transfer to an airtight container and store in the fridge for up to a week. You can also store the pesto in the freezer for up to 6 months.

Makes about 1 cup

¼ cup toasted pine nuts (see Tip in Caper-Currant Relish, page 25)

2 large cloves garlic, roughly chopped

¼ teaspoon kosher sea salt

2 packed cups fresh basil leaves (about 2½ ounces)

½ cup extra-virgin olive oil

2 tablespoons nutritional yeast

1 tablespoon freshly squeezed lemon juice

Swap It
Substitute toasted walnuts or pumpkin seeds for the pine nuts.

Tip
For extra sweetness and complexity, add 2 tablespoons of dried currants or raisins. For more creaminess and healthy fats, add half an avocado.

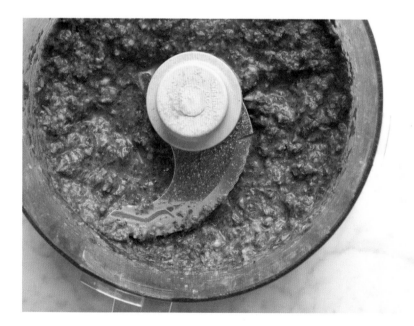

Creamy Thai Pesto

So the truth about how this sauce came to be goes like this: I tried 100 different ways of making an allergen-free pad thai–style sauce and it never really hit the spot. Pad thai is special. Sometimes substituting or omitting ingredients doesn't work when you're navigating the allergen-free-recipe waters. Often, I'd rather go in a completely different direction. While I was in the midst of testing other fresh green sauces and pestos, I decided to experiment with some Thai flavors and voilà! Holy moly. This is so unexpected and delightful—a simultaneously sweet-and-savory fusion of flavors that still tastes bright and fresh. The secret pantry ingredient here is dried shrimp. It's worth making a special trip to your local Asian market for this, or you can order it online. There are many kinds of dried shrimp, so look for the tiny wild ones that are about the size of a thumbnail (sometimes labeled "S" for their small size), usually sold in the refrigerated section of larger markets.

This sauce is super versatile. Try it on my Creamy Pad Thai Kelp Noodles (page 117), or spoon it over my Whole Roasted Branzino (page 151). You could also use it as a dipping sauce for Whole Garlic Prawns with Charred Lemon (page 159).

Pulse everything except the olive oil in a food processor until broken down into a thick paste. Scrape down the sides of the processor with a spatula, add ¼ cup of the olive oil, and pulse a few times, until a thick, creamy sauce has formed. Scrape down the sides again, add the remaining ¼ cup oil, and pulse again until well incorporated.

Use immediately, or transfer to an airtight container and store in the fridge for a week.

Makes about 1 cup

1 packed cup fresh basil leaves

1 packed cup fresh cilantro (with stems)

¼ cup creamy almond butter or peanut butter

¼ cup chopped green onions

3 tablespoons dried shrimp (wild, if available)

1 tablespoon plus 1 teaspoon coconut sugar

1 tablespoon lime zest

1 tablespoon lime juice

1 large clove garlic, roughly chopped

1 teaspoon minced fresh ginger

1 teaspoon fish sauce

Pinch of kosher sea salt

½ cup extra-virgin olive oil, divided

Tip

If you're allergic to nuts, you can substitute sunflower seed butter for the nut butter. If you're allergic to shrimp, simply omit and add 1 tablespoon of chickpea miso.

Cheesy Garlic Croutons

It's been a while since I was able to enjoy a cheesy, garlicky crouton like this one, which doesn't have gluten or dairy. You'll need a country-style loaf of bread for this recipe (like the Grain-Free Vegan Boule on page 201). Nutritional yeast, coupled with ghee, garlic, and herbs, helps create an incredible substitute for this classic staple. I've used fresh parsley here, but you could also use a teaspoon of dried parsley, oregano, or thyme instead.

Preheat the oven to 375°F, and line a large baking sheet with parchment paper.

Put the bread cubes in a large mixing bowl.

Heat a small saucepan over medium, and add the ghee and garlic. Gently sauté for 30 seconds, until fragrant, then turn off the heat.

Pour the garlic ghee over the croutons, add the parsley, nutritional yeast, salt, and pepper and mix gently with a rubber spatula until the bread cubes are fully coated with everything.

Transfer the croutons to the baking sheet and spread them out evenly in a single layer. Toast for 18 to 20 minutes, or until golden brown and crisp (no stirring necessary).

Remove from the oven and allow to cool completely for about an hour. The croutons will become crispier during this final step. Serve immediately, or store at room temperature in a bowl covered with a dish towel.

Makes about 4 cups

4 cups (½-inch) country-style gluten-free bread cubes (from about half a loaf of the Grain-Free Vegan Boule on page 201)

¼ cup ghee

2 large cloves garlic, minced

1 tablespoon minced fresh flat-leaf parsley

2 tablespoons nutritional yeast

Kosher sea salt

Freshly ground black pepper

Swap It
For a vegan version, you can substitute extra-virgin olive oil for the ghee. Garlic Confit oil (page 18) would be delicious here too, if you have some on hand. You can also use any country-style store-bought bread here as well.

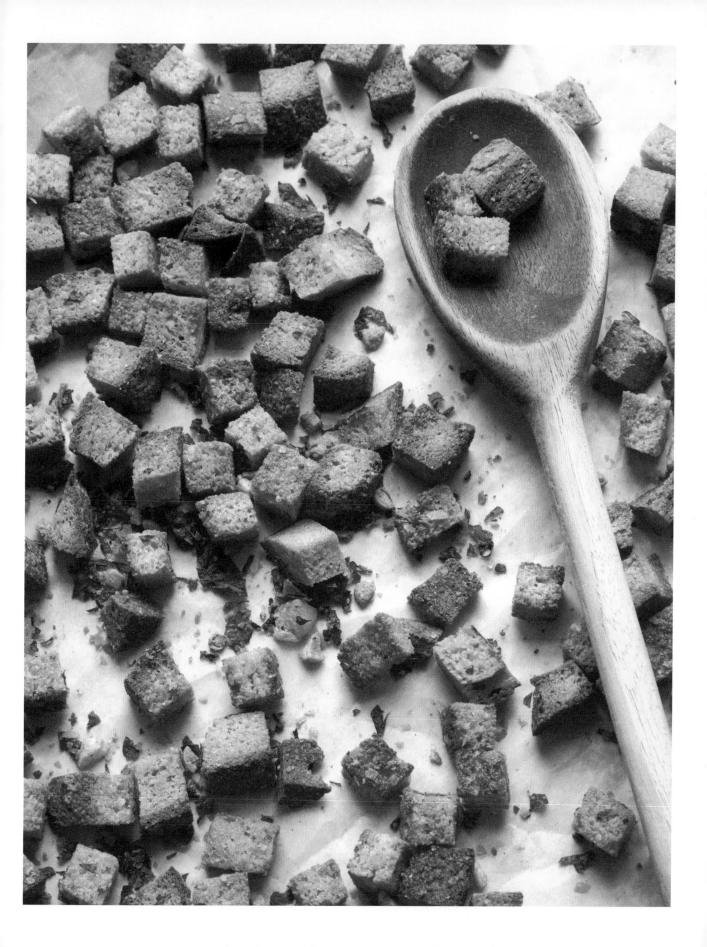

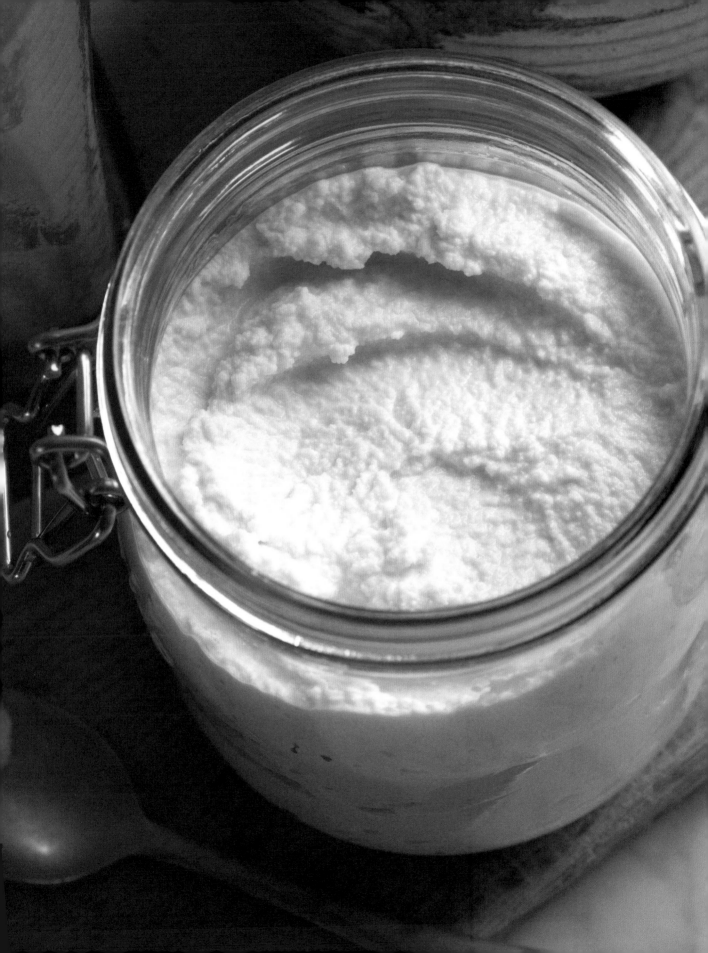

Fresh Almond Ricotta Cheese

My dear Greek friend Amalia introduced this cheese to me when she came to visit us in 2019. Honestly, I'm not one for processed vegan cheese made with gums, starches, soy, and peas . . . I'd rather pass altogether! But THIS cheese was a revelation. It's fresh, thick, and creamy, and it comes together quite easily. It's very versatile, a blank canvas that you can take in sweet or savory directions, making it perfect for pizza, pasta, dessert, and more! Make it as is, spread it on toast, and drizzle with Cherry Tomato Confit (page 18), or serve it on its own with fruit compote for a healthy breakfast. You can put it in lasagna, drop a dollop into your spaghetti, or blend it with fresh herbs. If you don't eat dairy, and you're looking for something to scratch that itch, look no further.

On your countertop, soak the almonds overnight in enough cold water to cover them.

The following day, drain and rinse the almonds and remove the skins by gently pinching them between your fingers.

Transfer the almonds to a high-speed upright blender. Add the water, lemon juice, and the salt. Blend until the mixture becomes thick and coarse, scraping down the sides if necessary. (It may take a moment to begin to move in the blender.) Add more water 1 tablespoon at a time until the cheese becomes almost smooth and creamy.

Transfer the cheese to an airtight container and store in the fridge, where it will firm up in a few hours and keep for 5 days.

Makes about 3 cups

2 cups raw almonds

1¼ cups water, plus more as needed

1 teaspoon lemon juice

½ teaspoon kosher sea salt

Tips

For a firmer cheese, use only 1 cup of water. (It's delicious to blend in a handful of soft fresh herbs here as well.) Transfer to a sieve lined with cheesecloth set over a bowl to drain. You can twist the cloth to form a bundle and squeeze gently. Drain in the fridge for a few hours.

For a savory variation of the ricotta, add ½ cup of fresh chopped herbs like dill or parsley, or add 2 tablespoons of nutritional yeast for a richer cheese flavor. You could also add 1 teaspoon onion or garlic powder.

For a sweet variation of the ricotta, add ½ teaspoon rose or orange blossom water, vanilla bean powder, citrus zest, or a combination of 2 tablespoons maple syrup and 1 teaspoon of alcohol-free vanilla extract.

Swap It

You can substitute the whole raw almonds with slivered almonds. In that case, soak them for just 30 minutes in hot water instead.

Fresh Almond Cream

This fresh almond cream is super simple and completely worth making from scratch. Its velvety, creamy texture makes it an ideal substitute for thick dairy cream. I use it in hot drinks and as an addition to soups and sauces. It's silky, with very little almond flavor, and very concentrated, so a little goes a long way. It's the perfect alternative creamer without all the junk.

Place the almonds in a mixing bowl, add boiling water to cover, and soak for 30 minutes. Drain, rinse, and transfer the almonds to an upright blender with the cold water.

Process for about 45 seconds on high speed, or until the mixture is velvety smooth and resembles cream.

Strain through a nut bag (or a fine-mesh strainer lined with a layer of cheesecloth), squeezing gently to press out all the cream, into a large measuring cup so you can easily transfer to an airtight container. Store in the fridge for up to a week.

Makes about 2 cups

1 cup slivered almonds
Boiling water
1½ cups cold water

Confit Three Ways

Having a jar of confit around is like having money in the bank. Confiting is a stealthy old-school French cooking technique that's a method of preservation. Meat and vegetables are typically slow-cooked in pure animal fat or olive oil, which preserves them and gives them tons of flavor, and also allows them to be stored safely for a few weeks in the fridge. This process allows you to prep ahead and build up a well-stocked "pantry" for future meals or to preserve ingredients that may no longer be in season. This is one of those moments when you serve your allergen-friendly meals and watch your loved ones squeal with joy as they devour your "special food."

I use a roughly 7-inch oval baking dish for my shallot and tomato confits (and a slightly smaller one for the garlic), but you could use anything, as long as the ingredients are submerged or almost submerged in the oil. Note that the oil in the confits will solidify in the fridge. Don't freak out—just dig out what you need or leave the jar at room temperature for about 30 minutes and it will reliquefy.

Shallot Confit

This is a beautiful condiment that can be spooned over sliced steak, folded into the Flatbreads dough (page 194), or whisked into salad dressing.

Preheat the oven to 300°F.

Place all the ingredients in a shallow baking dish and cover with enough olive oil to submerge the shallots at least three-quarters of the way. Roast for 1½ hours, or until the shallots are golden and fork-tender.

Remove from the oven and allow to cool completely. Transfer to a sealed container with the oil, and store in the fridge for up to 2 weeks.

Recipe continues

Makes about 4 cups

2 pounds shallots, peeled and halved

6 fresh thyme sprigs

3 fresh bay leaves

2 cups extra-virgin olive oil, or as needed

Garlic Confit

This sweet and versatile condiment can be used in numerous ways. You can add the garlic to soft butter or ghee, fold it into anything smashed, smear it over toast, blend it into soups or dips, spoon it over roasted vegetables, or use the scented oil in vinaigrette.

Preheat the oven to 300°F.

Place the garlic in a small, shallow baking dish, and add the thyme and bay leaves. Pour over enough olive oil to submerge the garlic at least a third of the way. Roast for 45 minutes, or until the garlic is light golden and tender.

Allow to cool completely, transfer to an airtight container with the oil, and store in the fridge for up to 2 weeks.

Makes about 2 cups

4 heads of garlic, cloves peeled

5 fresh thyme sprigs

2 fresh bay leaves

1 cup extra-virgin olive oil, or as needed

Cherry Tomato Confit

This sweet and luscious confit is perfect spooned over ricotta and toast, flatbreads, vegetables, sliced steak, fish, eggs, grains, or beans.

Preheat the oven to 300°F.

Place the tomatoes in a shallow baking dish. Tuck in the 2 half heads of garlic, scatter the thyme and basil on top, and sprinkle with salt. Pour over enough olive oil to submerge the tomatoes at least three-quarters of the way, tucking in the herbs as necessary. Roast for 1½ hours, or until the tomatoes are blistered and bubbling. (Larger tomatoes may take up to an extra hour.)

Allow to cool completely, then transfer to an airtight container with the oil and store in the fridge for up to 2 weeks. (Depending on how much you like garlic, you can squeeze out the garlic cloves and add them to the jar, too, or discard the garlic entirely.)

Makes about 6 cups

4 cups small cherry tomatoes

1 head of garlic, halved horizontally

6 fresh thyme sprigs

3 stems of basil leaves

½ teaspoon kosher sea salt

2 cups extra-virgin olive oil, or as needed

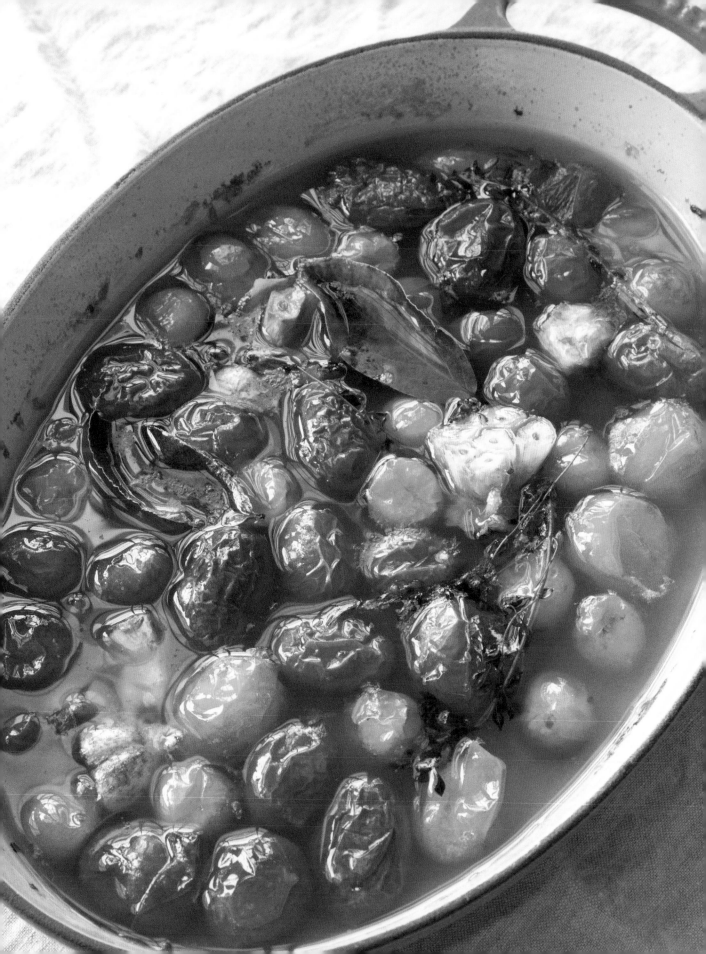

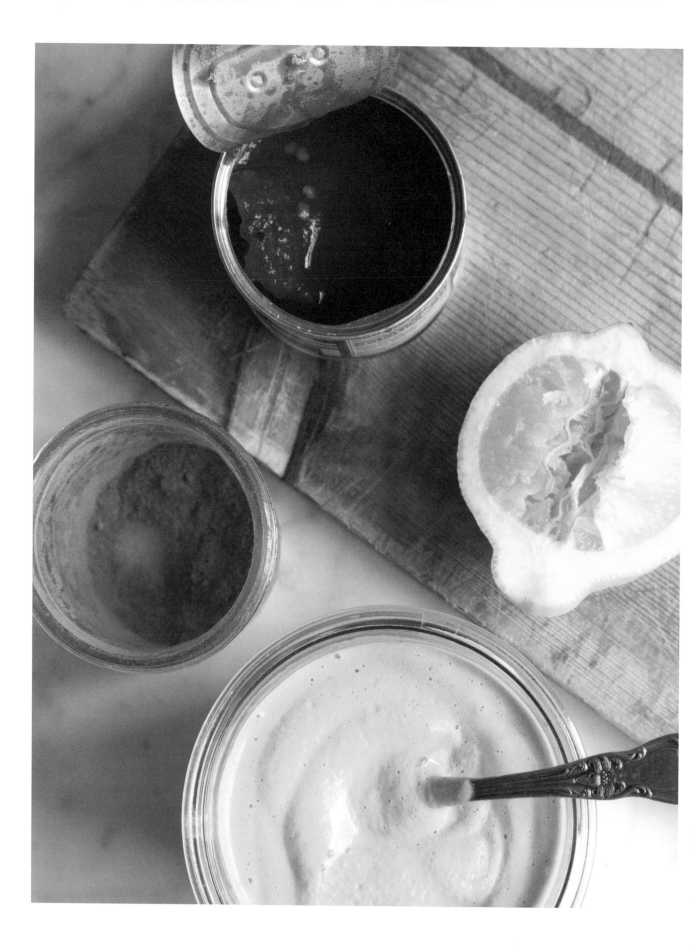

Chipotle Aioli

Creamy, spicy, smoky, sweet, and earthy—this sauce has it all! In the past, I've typically relied on cashews to make great mayonnaise, but I've steered away from cashews lately. (My doctor mentioned I should omit them from my diet for now, as they are related to the poison ivy family and can be irritating for some folks. Who knew?!) So I used slivered almonds here, instead, as a base to make this vegan condiment, and it is delicious. This sauce is perfect to drizzle over fish tacos or as a dipping sauce for fries, wings, or fritters. If you prefer cashews, you can use the same amount instead of almonds.

Place the almonds in a bowl and add boiling water to cover. Allow to soak for 30 minutes.

Drain and rinse the almonds, then transfer them to a high-speed upright blender. Add all the other ingredients and blend until smooth and creamy, about 1 minute. You may need to use a tamper or rubber spatula to help move things along if the mixture is too thick in the beginning. If you need to add more water, do so 1 tablespoon at a time. Adjust with lemon juice, salt, and maple syrup to your liking.

Use immediately, or transfer the sauce to an airtight container and store in the fridge for up to a week.

Makes about 2 cups

1 cup slivered almonds

Boiling water

¾ cup cold water, plus more

2 whole canned chipotle peppers in adobo sauce

2 tablespoons extra-virgin olive oil

1 small clove garlic, grated

1 tablespoon apple cider vinegar

1 teaspoon fresh lemon juice

1 teaspoon country-style Dijon mustard

2 teaspoons maple syrup

¼ teaspoon kosher sea salt

¼ teaspoon paprika

Tip
To make a plain mayonnaise, simply omit the chipotle peppers, garlic, and paprika.

Smashed Cumin Guacamole

Many years ago our annual holiday party featured a fully catered taco bar and an all-female mariachi band. It was awesome, except that the caterer got smashed and proceeded to flirt with half our guests, making a complete fool of himself. The next day he came back to apologize, and I told him we'd let him off the hook if he shared his secret guacamole recipe with me. He did. Inspired by his proportions, this recipe emerged, simplified. I left out the nightshades, used red onions instead of white, and added a dash of cumin. I've been making this dip for over a decade and people always notice the special spice. Like all simple dishes, it's important to pay attention to the details. Make sure your avocados are ripe but firm. You don't want mush; you want a sturdy dip that's still creamy.

I serve this with Mary's Gone Crackers and a big plate of crunchy fresh vegetables like cucumbers, radishes, and celery for those of us avoiding grains.

Cube the avocados, place them in a medium bowl, and add the lime juice and salt. Using a fork, smash the avocados until the mixture is creamy, with some larger-size chunks. Add the rest of the ingredients and mix well.

Transfer to a serving bowl. Serve immediately, or place in an airtight container and press a piece of plastic wrap over the surface of the guacamole, gently pushing out all the air. Then cover and refrigerate for up to 3 days.

Serves 6 to 8

4 Hass avocados, halved and pitted

1 tablespoon freshly squeezed lime juice

½ teaspoon kosher sea salt

¼ cup roughly chopped fresh cilantro

¼ cup finely minced red onion

½ teaspoon ground cumin

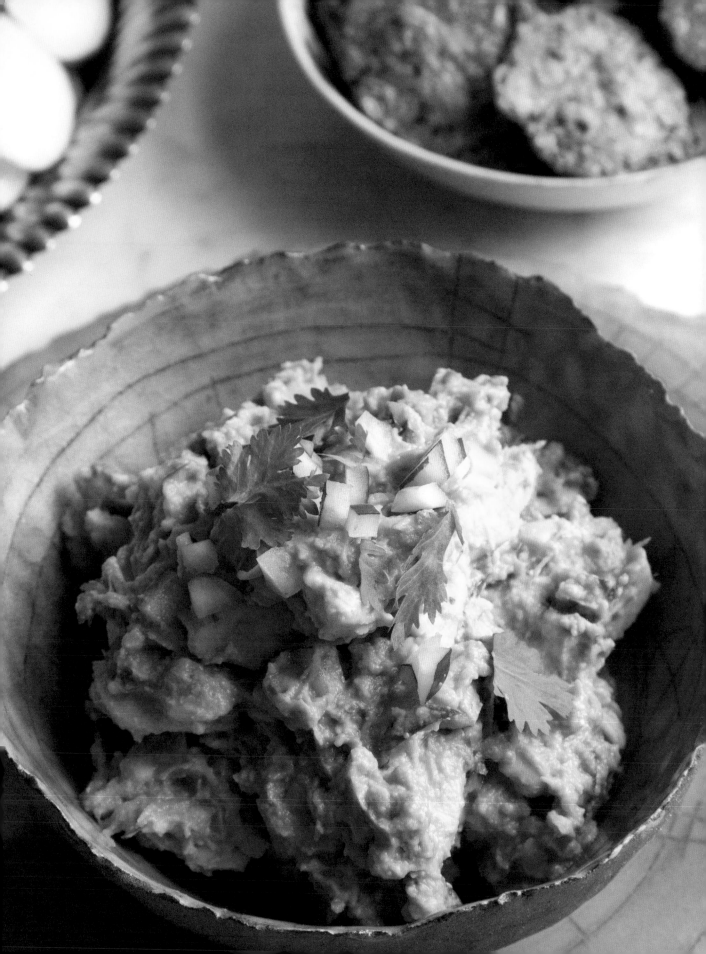

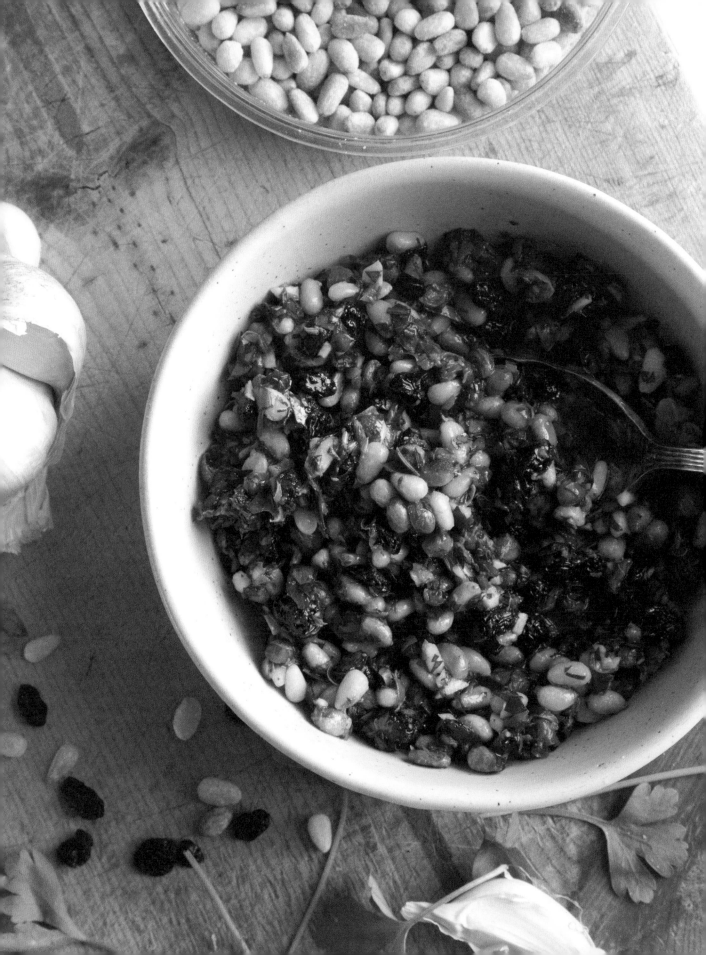

Caper-Currant Relish

I developed this relish with the Pan-Roasted Cauliflower (page 128) in mind, but you can spoon this delicious condiment over most roasted vegetables, fish, and poultry. I would also be happy to eat this on toasted garlic bread with olive oil. It's a lovely combination of sweet-and-sour ingredients with soft toasty nuts, punchy acids, and fresh herbs. It feels like the zestier and livelier cousin of *agrodolce*—the one who comes into town ready to party. You might want to double the recipe because it disappears fast.

In a medium mixing bowl, combine all the ingredients and stir gently until everything is mixed well. Taste and adjust seasoning. Allow the flavors to develop for at least 10 minutes.

Use immediately, or transfer to an airtight container and store in the fridge for up to a week.

Makes about ¾ cup

¼ cup toasted pine nuts

¼ cup dried currants

3 tablespoons extra-virgin olive oil

3 tablespoons finely chopped flat-leaf parsley

2 tablespoons capers, rinsed and finely chopped

1 teaspoon lemon zest

1 tablespoon freshly squeezed lemon juice

1 tablespoon sherry vinegar

1 large clove garlic, finely chopped

1 teaspoon maple syrup

Kosher sea salt

Freshly ground black pepper

Tips

To toast pine nuts, simply warm them in a small, dry nonstick skillet over medium heat, shaking the pan occasionally to ensure they don't burn, 2 to 3 minutes. Transfer them to a plate to cool.

You can mix this relish with a jar of oil-packed wild tuna fish, drained of excess oil, for an impromptu tuna salad to eat on its own or spoon over toast.

Sticky Plum BBQ Sauce

This is my answer to a nightshade-free barbecue sauce, which means it can't rely on tomato, like most sauces do. There are many "nomato" sauces out there that mix carrots and beets together to produce a tomato-like sauce alternative for those of us avoiding nightshades. I've never gravitated toward them because those flavors feel too earthy to me, especially when I think of tomatoes, which are sweet and tart. I decided to look for inspiration from Asian cuisine instead, and landed on the sweet, dark, and tart flavors of plum jam. This lays a beautiful and sticky foundation to build on with tamari, fish sauce, spices, and fresh aromatics. It blends into a sweet-and-savory barbecue sauce for ribs, chicken, and vegetables. If you're avoiding soy, see Swap It for a delicious substitute.

In a medium saucepan over medium heat, add all the ingredients, stirring together, and bring to a gentle boil. Then simmer on low for 5 minutes, or until the aromatics are soft.

Transfer to an upright blender and mix on high for 30 seconds, or until all the aromatics have broken down and the sauce is smooth and thick. Use immediately, or transfer to an uncovered airtight container to cool, then cover and refrigerate for up to 2 weeks.

Makes about 2 cups

1 cup plum jam (such as Bonne Maman Plum Preserves)

4 cloves garlic, roughly chopped

1-inch piece fresh ginger, peeled and roughly chopped

¼ cup minced green onion (from about 1 stalk)

1 teaspoon Chinese five-spice powder

1 tablespoon apple cider vinegar

¼ cup plus 2 tablespoons tamari

1 tablespoon fish sauce

¼ cup water

Swap It
To make this soy-free, you can substitute coconut aminos for the tamari and add an extra tablespoon each of fish sauce and apple cider vinegar.

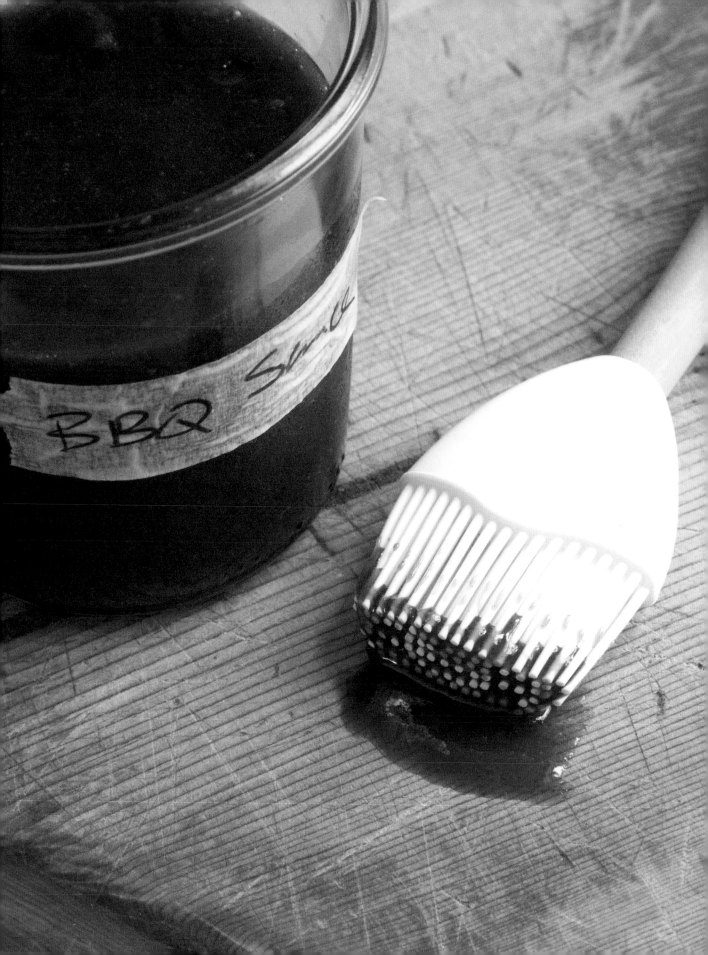

Quick Pickles

Give me bright, tangy, zippy, crunchy veg and I'll find something to add them to at any time of day. We pile them into every kind of taco, drop them into salads, tuck them into sandwiches, use them to top off bean bowls, or pile them onto a crudités board, but you can also just snack on pickles (which are super easy to make) whenever. I've included three different types of vinegar you can use to play around with and some spices that work nicely, too. This is very forgiving, so have fun with it—you can't go wrong.

Quick Pickled Red Onions

Place the vinegar in a small saucepan with the honey, salt, fennel, coriander, and bay leaf. Gently cook for a few minutes on medium-low heat, stirring, until the salt dissolves. Turn off the heat and let the mixture cool for 10 minutes.

Put the onions in a medium bowl and pour the brine mixture over them. Toss everything by hand, and make sure all the vegetables are saturated. Allow to cure for 15 minutes, then transfer to a glass jar or storage container along with the brine.

Enjoy immediately, or store in the fridge for up to 2 weeks.

Makes about 1½ cups

½ cup champagne vinegar

4 teaspoons honey

2 teaspoons kosher sea salt

1 teaspoon fennel seeds

1 teaspoon coriander seeds

1 dried bay leaf

1 medium red onion, thinly sliced (about 2 cups)

Quick Pickled Radishes

Place the vinegar in a small saucepan with the honey and salt. Gently cook for a few minutes on medium-low heat, stirring, until the salt dissolves. Turn off the heat and let the mixture cool for 10 minutes.

Put the radishes in a medium bowl and pour the brine mixture over them. Toss everything by hand, and make sure all the radishes are saturated. Allow to cure for 15 minutes, then transfer to a glass jar or storage container along with the brine.

Makes about 1½ cups

½ cup rice vinegar

2 teaspoons honey

2 teaspoons kosher sea salt

½ pound radishes, thinly sliced (about 2 cups)

Quick Pickled Cucumbers

Place the vinegar in a small saucepan with the honey, salt, dill seed, and garlic. Gently cook for a few minutes on medium-low heat, stirring, until the salt dissolves. Turn off the heat and let the mixture cool for 10 minutes.

Put the cucumbers in a medium bowl and pour the brine mixture over them. Toss everything by hand, and make sure all the cucumbers are saturated. Allow to cure for 15 minutes, then transfer to a glass jar or storage container along with the brine.

Makes about 1½ cups

½ cup apple cider vinegar

2 teaspoons honey

2 teaspoons kosher sea salt

1 teaspoon dill seed or celery seed

2 cloves garlic, smashed

½ pound Persian cucumbers, thinly sliced (about 2 cups)

Tip
Peppers, carrots, fennel, green beans, asparagus, or cauliflower can all be quick pickled. Experiment with the vegetables you like, cutting larger, sturdier vegetables into smaller pieces so they soften more easily in the brine.

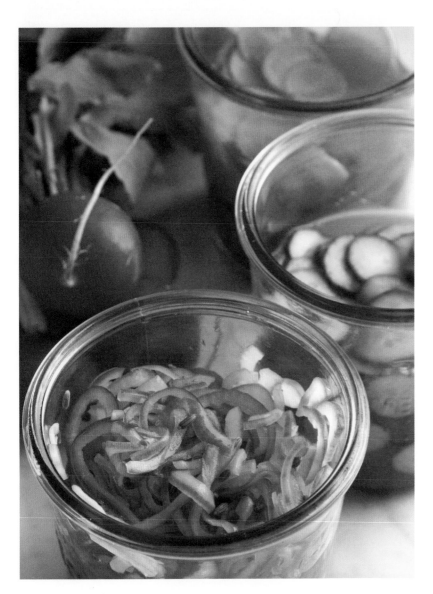

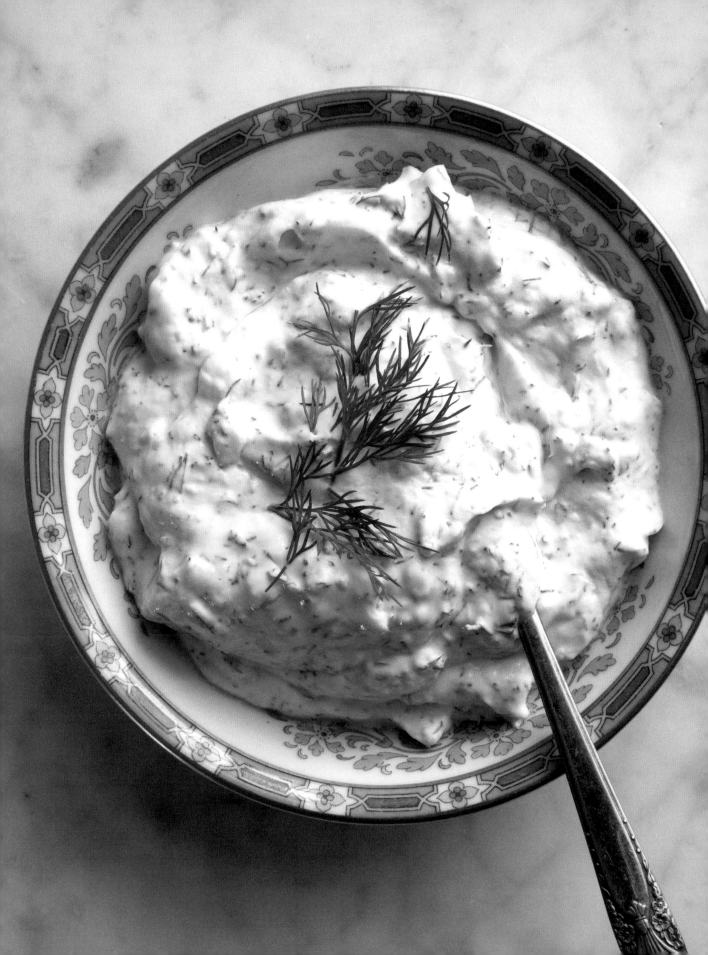

Coconut Yogurt Tzatziki

Part of the journey with using alternative ingredients is learning how to experiment with flavors and textures so that you can achieve a familiar and joyful eating experience. When you get the balance right for this sauce, it is such a treat! But it's important to use a thick Greek-style coconut yogurt. Before you start this recipe, go hunting for the best, thickest coconut yogurt you can find. If your yogurt is thin, strain it in a cheesecloth-lined sieve set over a bowl in the fridge for about an hour, or until it has thickened, before beginning. Coconut yogurts can vary, so I encourage you to taste it and balance the flavors to your liking. You may need to add more lemon, maple syrup, or salt.

Serve as a dip, a dollop, or a sandwich spread, or drizzle over fish tacos.

In a medium bowl, combine all the ingredients and whisk together. Taste and adjust to your liking.

Transfer to an airtight storage container and refrigerate for up to a week.

Makes about 1 cup

1 cup unsweetened, plain Greek-style coconut yogurt (such as Cocojune Pure Coconut)

1 small clove garlic, grated

1 teaspoon lemon zest

Juice of half a small lemon

¼ cup finely chopped fresh dill

1 teaspoon maple syrup

¼ teaspoon kosher sea salt

Freshly ground black pepper (optional)

Swap It
To make this a coconut-lime crema, substitute finely chopped cilantro for the dill and swap lime zest and juice for the lemon. It would be great on Wild Fried Fish Tacos (page 156).

You can also play around with other fresh herbs like parsley and chives, or add ½ teaspoon of spices like cumin, paprika, or curry powder. You can also omit the dill and add ¼ cup freshly grated horseradish for a spicy sauce to accompany steak.

Vanilla Berry Compote

Who needs store-bought jam when you can whip up a batch of fresh compote at home in less than 30 minutes? Unlike preserves, compote is meant to be used straightaway. It also has larger whole chunks of fruit in it, making it less spreadable and more of a hearty, luscious topping. I smother this all over my pancakes, mix it with yogurt, or layer it with smashed cookies and Fresh Almond Ricotta Cheese for a heavenly home-made dessert.

In a medium pot over medium heat, melt the ghee. Add the strawberries, maple syrup, lemon juice, and vanilla. Cook, stirring occasionally, until the berries begin to release their juices, about 5 minutes. Once the juices release, simmer, stirring frequently, until the berries soften, 10 to 15 minutes more.

Leave as is or mash with a wooden spoon for a more muddled texture. Cool and transfer to a glass jar, cover, and store in the fridge for a week.

Makes about 2 cups

2 tablespoons ghee

1 pound (about 3 cups) trimmed and halved strawberries

2 tablespoons maple syrup

1 teaspoon lemon juice

1 teaspoon alcohol-free vanilla extract

Swap It
Substitute any kind of berry for the strawberries. Frozen berries work well, too.

Substitute coconut oil or butter for the ghee.

Substitute orange juice for the lemon juice.

Tip
Add a dash of ground cinnamon, ground cardamom, or rose water.

Spiced Toasted Seeds

Toasting seeds brings out their oils and intensifies their flavor. Paired with various herbs and spices, they get transformed from a simple ingredient to almost a dish of their own. They also become extra crunchy, making them an ideal topping. You can go sweet or savory and play around with different spices, herbs, sweeteners, or oils. During the holiday season, they make lovely gifts, too: roast a few large trays of these seeds, transfer them to labeled mason jars, and let your inner Martha Stewart go wild!

Za'atar Toasted Pepitas

Za'atar is a Middle Eastern spice mix that traditionally combines thyme, sesame seeds, and sumac. There are, of course, many variations of this blend, and the result is something of a woodsy, floral, nutty, and tangy situation. I first experienced this seasoning at a pub in the English countryside, where they served it heavily sprinkled over fresh house-made hummus with loads of warm pita. I like to toss these roasted homemade pepitas with this unique spice blend to create a complex, crunchy topping to use over salads, soups, dips, and vegetables.

Preheat the oven to 350°F, and line a large baking sheet with parchment paper.

In a small bowl, combine all the spices and the salt and mix.

In a medium bowl, add the pepitas, olive oil, and spice mixture and toss thoroughly by hand. Pour them onto the baking sheet and spread them out evenly in a single layer.

Roast for 15 to 20 minutes, stirring the pepitas halfway through cooking to help them brown evenly.

Remove from the oven and allow to cool for about an hour. Transfer to an airtight container and store at room temperature for about 2 weeks, or in the fridge for up to 2 months.

Makes about 2 cups

1 teaspoon dried thyme

1 teaspoon sesame seeds

1 teaspoon ground sumac

½ teaspoon kosher sea salt

2 cups raw pepitas (pumpkin seeds)

1 tablespoon extra-virgin olive oil

Swap It
Substitute dried marjoram or dried oregano for the dried thyme.

Toasted Maple Sunflower Seeds

When we lived in Upstate New York, we would sometimes visit the town of Great Barrington, Massachusetts, where our daughter briefly attended school. I loved visiting that town because of the inspiring restaurants and an amazing health-food store that was stocked with gorgeous local produce and meats. I went to the same restaurant every time and ordered the same simple green salad that was topped off with sweet and crunchy sunflower seeds. I needed to make my own version, and here they are! Throw a small handful of these over any fresh tossed salad, noodle bowl, or yogurt bowl, or just snack on them straight from the jar.

Preheat the oven to 350°F, and line a large baking sheet with parchment paper.

In a medium bowl, combine all the ingredients and mix well with a rubber spatula. Pour the seeds onto the prepared baking sheet and spread them out evenly into a single layer.

Roast for 12 to 15 minutes, or until golden brown.

Remove from the oven and allow to cool completely, about an hour. They will be stuck together like a brittle, so gently break them apart into pieces by scrunching them by hand directly on the pan. Transfer to an airtight container and store at room temperature for up to a month.

Makes about 2 cups

2 cups raw sunflower seeds

2 tablespoons maple syrup

1 tablespoon coconut sugar

1 teaspoon extra-virgin olive oil

¾ teaspoon kosher sea salt

Swap It
You can substitute honey for the maple syrup and melted coconut oil for the olive oil.

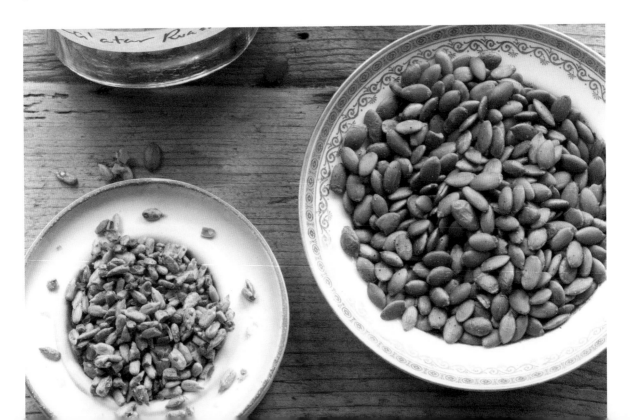

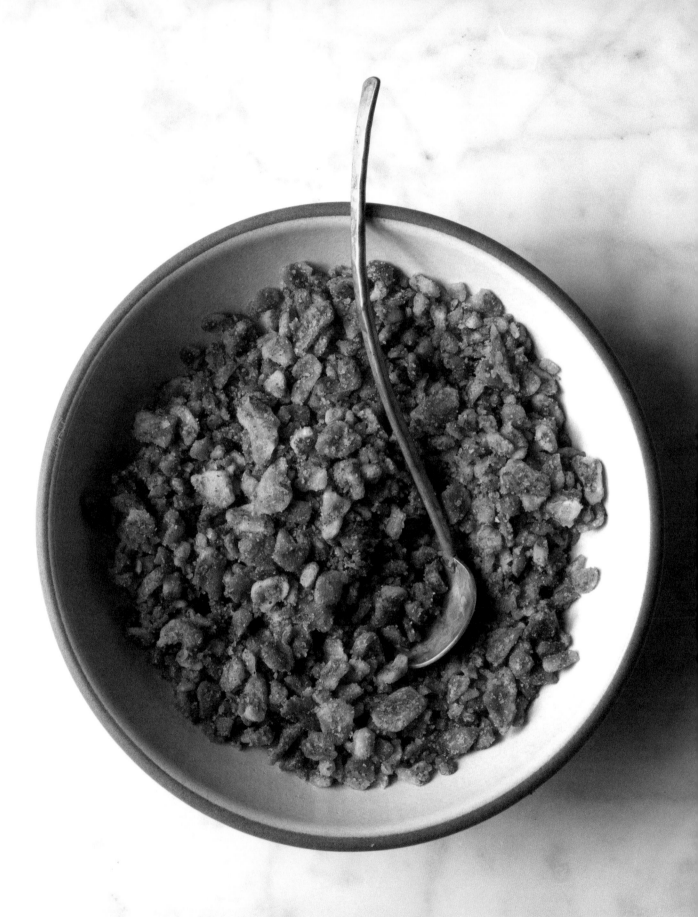

Toasted Plantain Crumbs

It is essential to find replacements for familiar flavors and textures when you want to make lasting and sustainable changes to your diet. Eating is sensual. We crave a variety of textures when we eat, and crunch is my favorite. If your diet is grain-free, it's harder to find crunch. For me, I need special crunchy moments to keep me excited and passionate about staying the course. Enter toasted plantain crumbs. While I love them, these crumbs also provide joy for the folks at my table who are not on any particular diet. This preparation is best for topping a salad with creamy dressing (page 73), garnishing a simple pasta dish (page 113), or sprinkling over caramelized roasted vegetables (page 122). If you're looking for more of a breading style of crumb, simply process the chips until they are finer and skip the toasting step altogether (see Tip).

Preheat the oven to 350°F, and line a rimmed baking sheet with parchment paper.

Empty the bag of chips into the bowl of a food processor and process until they resemble coarse crumbs, about 30 seconds.

Spread them out on the baking sheet and roast for 13 to 15 minutes, or until golden brown.

Remove from the oven and allow to cool completely, about an hour. This final step is important, as they will continue to crisp up.

Transfer to an airtight container and store at room temperature, where they will keep for up to 2 weeks.

Makes about 1 cup

1 (5-ounce) bag plain, salted plantain chips (such as Barnana Organic Plantain Chips)

Tip
For an Italian-style "breading," add ½ teaspoon of each or just some of the following dried herbs to the food processor with the chips before processing: oregano, thyme, basil, rosemary, marjoram, and/or sage.

Bone Broth

This is pure medicine. If you have any gut issues, drinking one to three cups of this broth a day can really help to heal and restore your microbiome and gut lining. But if you have a histamine intolerance, you should avoid bone broth.

This broth is full of vitamins, amino acids, and essential fatty acids that support the immune system, boost heart health, and help repair body tissue. I call it "liquid gold."

It's very important to try and source good-quality collagen-rich bones, like knuckle or marrow bones, that are from animals free of antibiotics and hormones. Many wonderful farms are practicing sustainable and regenerative farming techniques that do right by their animals and the land. If you can't find them locally, go online. They should be affordable and easy to find.

I've left out any spices and salt so you can use the broth in a multitude of ways. It's a rich neutral base for drinking or cooking. Feel free to season it to your liking.

Place all the ingredients in a multicooker or pressure cooker, then add water up to the fill line. Do not fill past the fill line. Lock the lid and cook on high pressure for 4 hours. (You can also cook in a slow cooker on the high setting for 24 hours.)

Allow the pot to depressurize naturally, about 30 minutes.

Let the broth cool for a few hours, until the cooking bowl is just warm to the touch, then strain the broth and transfer it into glass jars or other airtight containers and store in the fridge for up to 5 days. You can also freeze this for up to 6 months.

Makes about 3 quarts

3 pounds beef, chicken, lamb, or pork bones (preferably knuckle or marrow, but any bones will do)

1 large celery stalk

1 large carrot

1 large yellow onion, unpeeled, quartered

Half a head of garlic, smashed and unpeeled (5 to 7 cloves)

2 bay leaves (fresh or dried)

Handful of flat-leaf parsley (including stems)

3 tablespoons apple cider vinegar

2 to 3 quarts water

Tip

For a richer-flavored broth, you can roast the bones prior to cooking. Simply place them on a baking sheet in a 425°F oven and roast for about 45 minutes, or until browned. Add the browned bones to the multicooker with the other ingredients, along with any browned bits from the roasting pan.

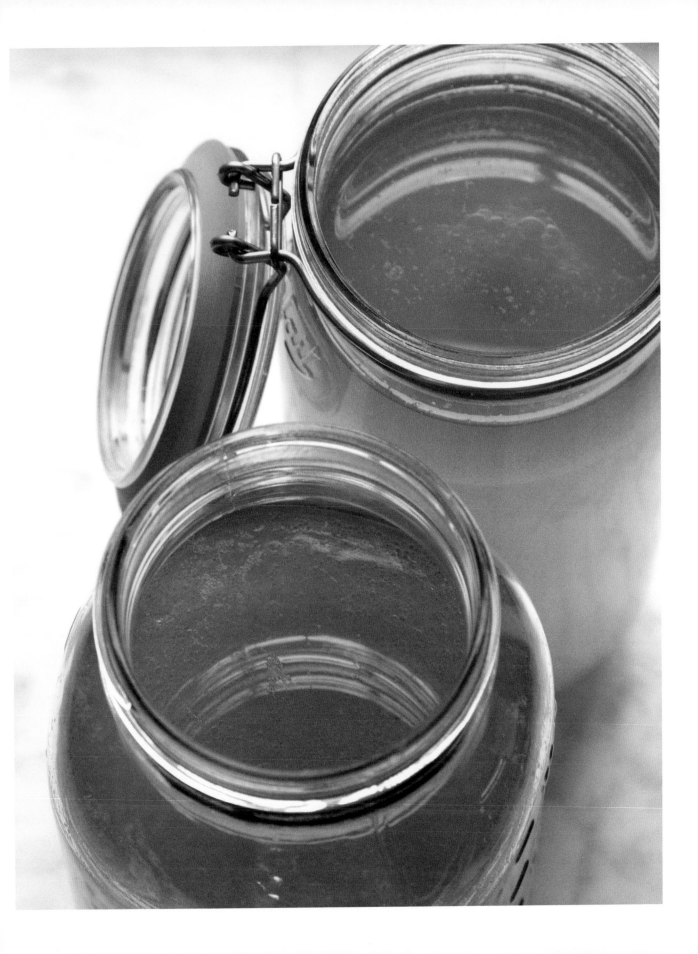

Big Batch of Beans

This is a super-simple and basic recipe for a cozy pot of deeply flavorful beans. Having a pot of beans on hand during the week sets you up for all kinds of delicious meals and supports your health with one of the most important nutrients we have in our diet: fiber. Fiber helps to remove toxins from the body and regulate your blood sugar. Beans have the most fiber of all foods. There's a lot of confusion out there about whether to soak beans. My reasoning for soaking beans has less to do with speeding up the cook time and more to do with gut health.

There is a belief that soaking beans prior to cooking helps to break down their lectins. Lectins are a family of protein found in most foods but especially beans, peanuts, grains, and nightshades. Some people believe that lectins can cause increased gut permeability and drive autoimmune disease. However, it is also believed that the soaking and cooking processes virtually eliminate lectins, making it safe to consume these foods if they are prepared properly.

Experiment and decide what works best for your body. But in my view, soaking beans is an easy and hands-off step that might help, certainly won't hurt, and speeds up cooking time—so why not do it?

You can also add spices like ground cumin or ground curry powder to change the flavor profile or chili peppers if you prefer heat. You can try adding half a lemon, a Parmesan rind, or a hunk of pancetta to the cooking liquid to enrich the beans even more.

In a big bowl, soak the dried beans in plenty of cold water (cover the beans by about 2 inches) and leave on the countertop overnight.

The following day, when you're ready to cook them, drain and rinse the beans and place them in a large Dutch oven or stockpot. Add all the other ingredients and cover with cold water by about 1½ inches. Bring to a gentle boil, then simmer until the beans are creamy and tender but not mushy. With a large spoon, skim off any foam that collects on the surface during cooking.

Serves 10

2½ cups dried beans (such as cannellini, black, pinto, kidney, or navy)

1 red onion, quartered through the root end

1 head of garlic, halved crosswise

3 fresh bay leaves

6 fresh thyme sprigs

1½ tablespoons kosher sea salt

¼ cup extra-virgin olive oil

Tip
You can serve these straight out of the pot alongside meat, chicken, fish, grains, or vegetables. You can add a few spoonfuls to your salad, toss them in a vinaigrette, mash them over toast, put them in tacos, add 1 pound of browned ground meat to the pot and make a spontaneous chili, or have them for breakfast with Beans, Greens + Broken Eggs (page 62).

Swap It
You can substitute rosemary, parsley, or sage for the thyme.

Cooking times can vary from 25 to 90 minutes, depending on the size of the beans and their freshness. Stir occasionally, tasting for doneness throughout the cooking process. The beans are done when they are soft and tender or creamy inside.

Add a little more water if its level drops below the surface of the beans; no more than an inch above the beans is necessary.

When the beans are done, remove from the heat and adjust seasoning. Serve immediately, or allow them to cool in their own liquid. Once cooled, remove and discard the aromatics and store the beans in their own liquid in the fridge for up to 5 days.

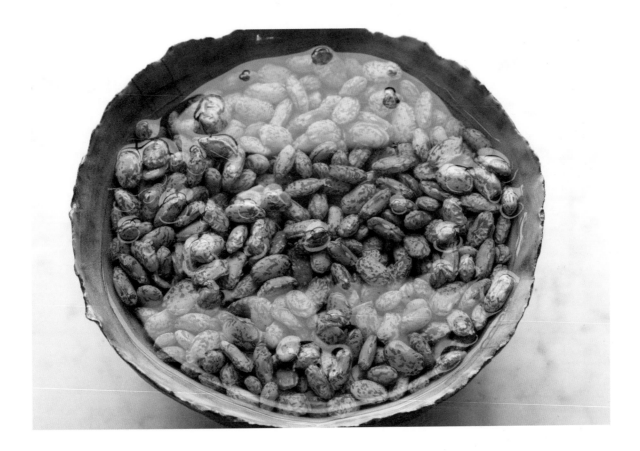

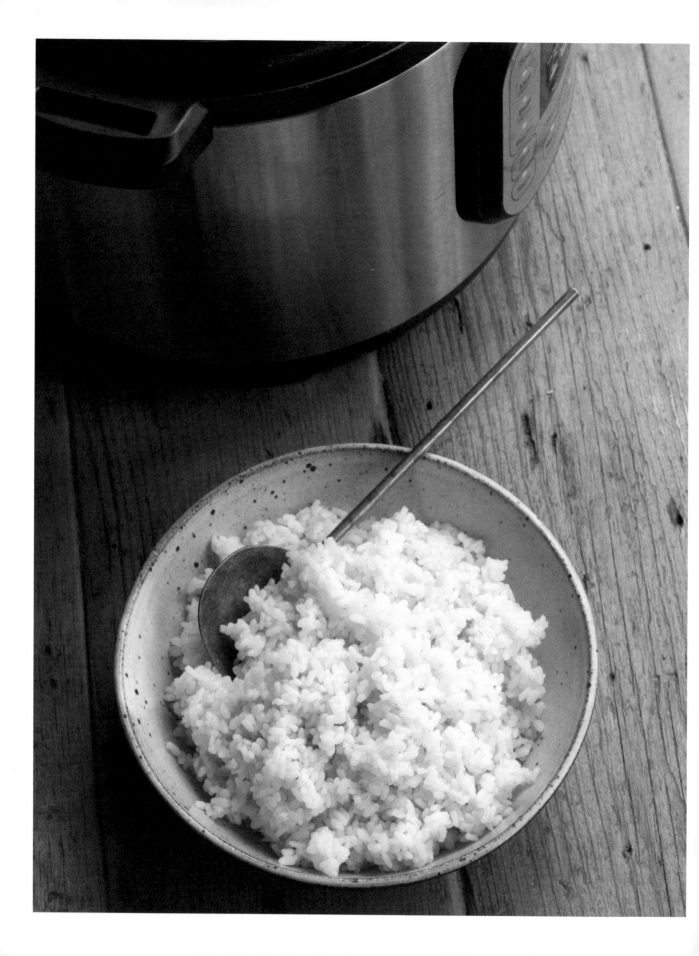

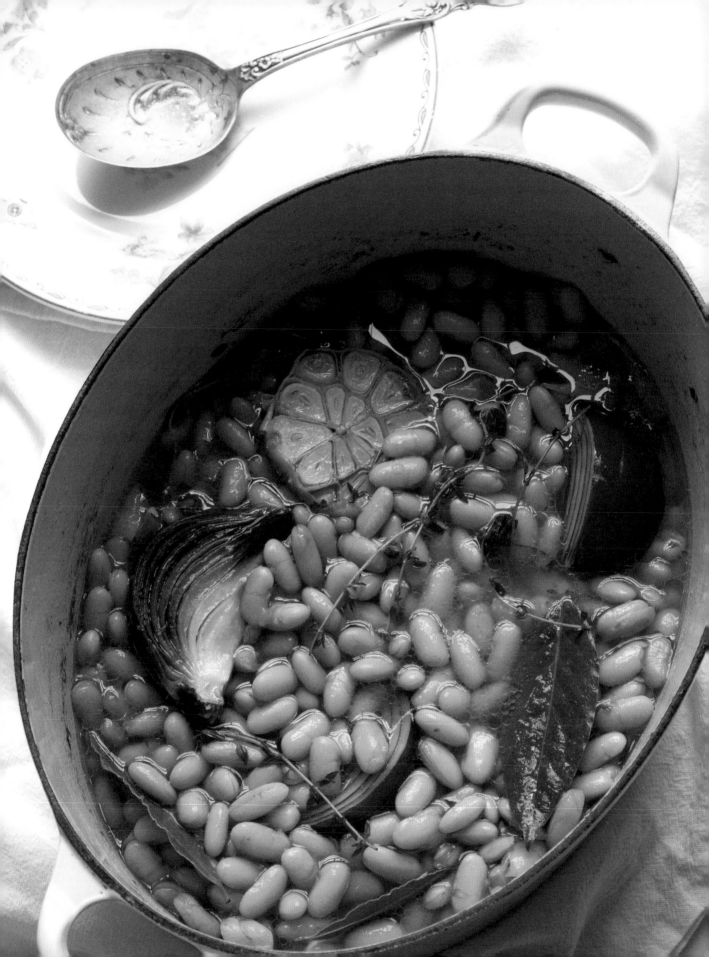

Big Batch of Short-Grain Rice

Why is it that rice can be so difficult to cook? There are many theories, but the one that makes the most sense to me is about evaporation. Depending on the pot that you use, and how well the lid seals in moisture, you may or may not struggle to achieve perfectly cooked rice with your favorite stove-top method. This is precisely why I *love* using a pressure cooker. (I use an Instant Pot, but any multicooker will do.) I get consistent, perfectly cooked rice every. single. time. There is something so completely divine about tender rice with just the right amount of tooth, similar to the pleasure of a just-right al dente pasta. I prefer short-grain rice over longer grains like jasmine or basmati because of its hearty chew. You can jazz it up with flavorful broth, aromatics, herbs, and spices—or you can enjoy it plain like we do, cooked in just water. Yup, no salt, nothing. This is a journey of purity and texture. It's also a beautiful backdrop for a delicious sauce and one of the easiest accompaniments to get on the table to round out a meal. With a pressure cooker or multicooker, you don't have to worry about it or keep a watchful eye on it. So relax into your life a little more deeply—this preparation has your back. Use this recipe to make a big batch of rice for the week (or for your next dinner party), knowing it will be perfect. It's also worth mentioning that pressure-cooking grains and beans has been shown to help break down their phytic acid and other anti-nutrients, helping them to be more easily digestible.

Lastly, it is said you must rinse your rice. I can't help you here. In cooking school, I learned that we should, but in real life I never do and nothing bad has ever happened. Ever. You decide.

Sushi Rice

Combine the rice and the water in the bowl of a multicooker. Swirl it around with a wooden spoon or your fingers, making sure all the rice is mixed well with the water. Give the bowl a little shake to even out the grains.

Lock the lid and make sure the pressure valve is sealed. Pressure-cook on high for 10 minutes, then let it release naturally for 10 minutes. Release the valve, unlock and remove the lid, and allow the rice to rest uncovered for a few minutes. Use a wooden spoon or rice paddle to fluff the rice, transfer it to a medium bowl, and serve immediately.

To store, allow the rice to cool, transfer to an airtight container, and refrigerate for up to a week.

Makes about 7 cups cooked rice

3 cups sushi rice

3 cups water

Short-Grain Brown Rice

Combine the rice and the water in the bowl of an Instant Pot. Swirl it around with a wooden spoon or your fingers, making sure all the rice is mixed well with the water. Give the bowl a little shake to even out the grains.

Lock the lid and make sure the pressure valve is sealed. Pressure-cook on high for 20 minutes, then let it release naturally for 10 minutes. Release the valve, unlock and remove the lid, and allow the rice to rest uncovered for 5 minutes. Use a wooden spoon or rice paddle to fluff the rice, transfer it to a medium bowl, and serve immediately.

To store, allow the rice to cool, transfer to an airtight container, and refrigerate for up to a week.

Makes about 7 cups cooked rice

3 cups short-grain brown rice

3¾ cups water

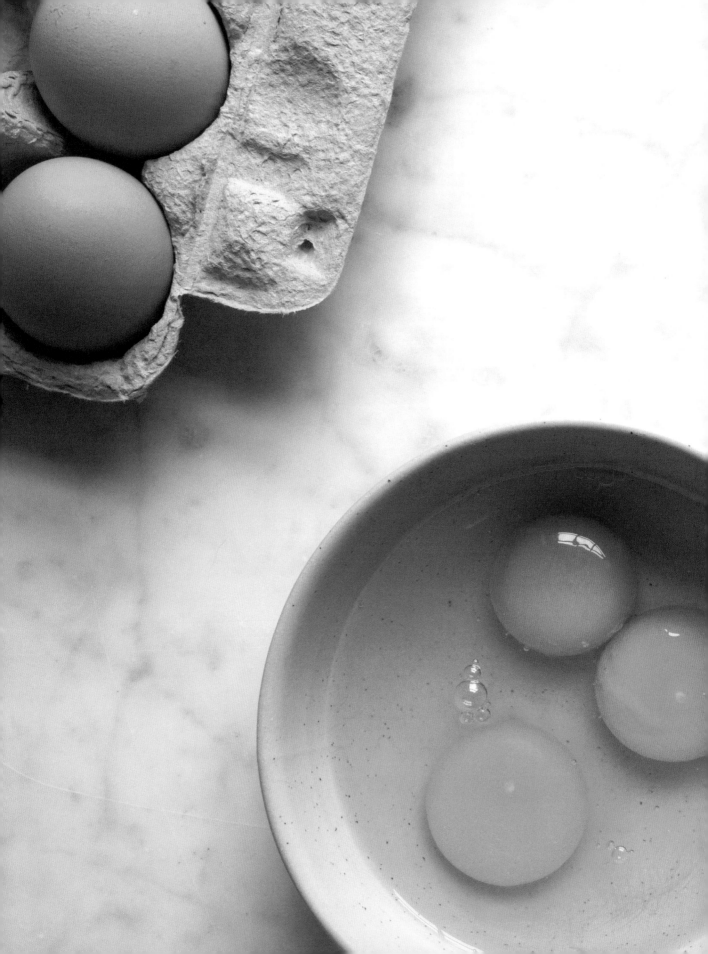

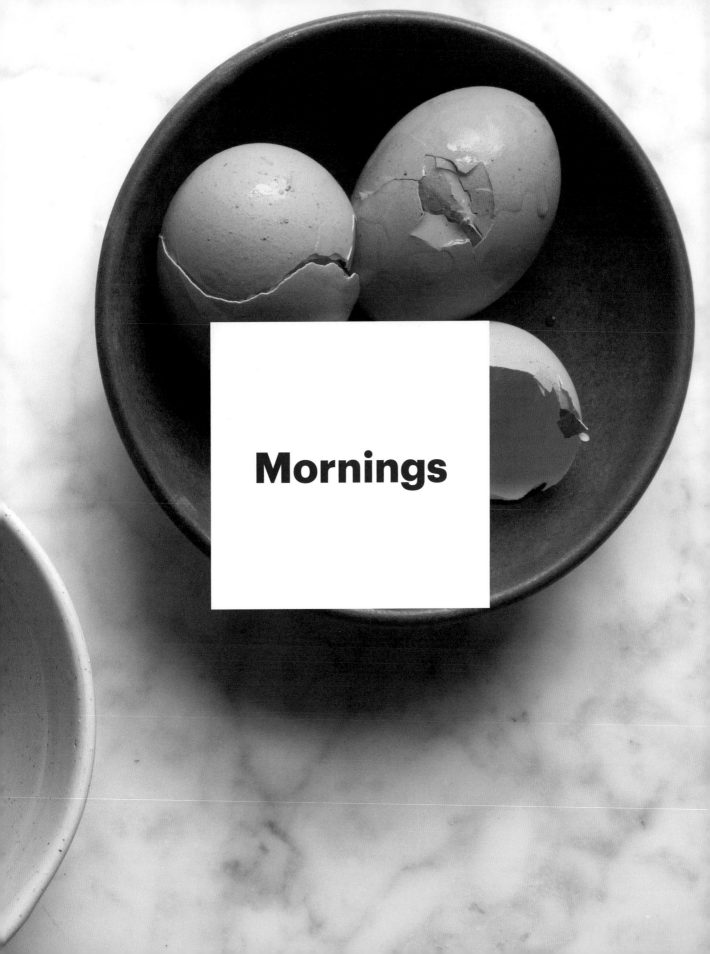

Mornings

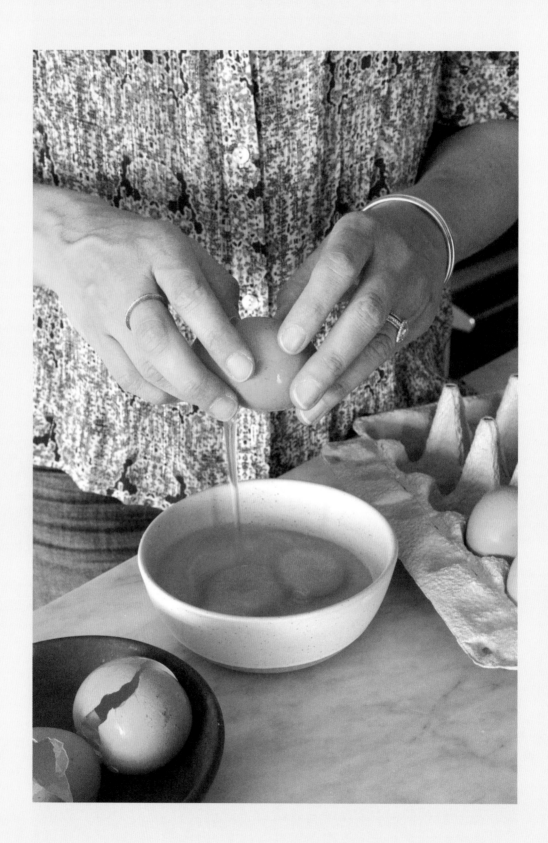

Food Is Love

Food is my love language. Watching someone savor a dish or a meal I've prepared is one of my greatest pleasures. As a host and a home cook, I'm always balancing my own dietary needs with what my guests like. Usually, I don't have to bend over backward to make different things for everyone at the table. But sometimes (especially at breakfast) I like to have fun with it and put in the extra effort; I try to remember what others love to eat and make sure to include their favorites at the dining table alongside my own.

I actually enjoy making some of the foods I no longer eat myself, because I still feel a connection to them through cooking. Take eggs, for example. I don't eat them anymore, but I love preparing them. Eggs are delicate and really require attention. I particularly love making poached, over-easy, and soft-scrambled eggs. Sometimes my in-laws come and visit for the weekend, and we have a house full of family with different eating styles. I usually assemble a robust Continental-style breakfast, complete with a gorgeous Grain-Free Vegan Boule I can eat and really enjoy (page 201). For the gluten-eating folks, I make sure to buy a beautiful loaf of regular hearty, fresh-baked bread and croissants. I get half-and-half and butter for the dairy eaters and make Fresh Almond Cream (page 16) for myself. I whip up a griddle full of over-easy eggs (which takes five minutes), and I put out a large tub of thick, plain unsweetened Greek-style vegan coconut yogurt with Vanilla Berry Compote (page 32) and Grain-Free Granola (page 54) that I usually have in the pantry.

We all come to the table with a unique set of circumstances and preferences, and this sort of spread includes everyone's favorites. This doesn't mean you have to become a short-order cook at every meal. It means that sometimes, with smart planning, you can assemble a simple, lovely meal that makes people—including yourself—feel extra welcome and loved.

Super Green Veg + Fruit Shake

When we lived in Los Angeles for 12 years, I fully embraced the Cali lifestyle. I adopted a mostly plant-based diet, had a few potted citrus trees on our patio, and juiced and cleansed on a regular basis. I learned a lot about my body during that time, and it wasn't until we moved back to the East Coast that I realized it wasn't in fact a good fit for me. I was tired a lot and just didn't feel grounded. Since then, I have discovered that I do much better with wild fish and pastured animal proteins, healthy fats, and lots of vegetables. I do still drink fresh-pressed juices and shakes, but I'm able to better customize them to my needs. A shake can be a deeply nourishing meal when it's balanced correctly. Remember that fruit is still sugar, so if you are trying to be moderate with sugar, don't load up on fruit-only shakes. You can pack a ton of fiber and phytonutrients in there with whole vegetables, too. Add a scoop of your favorite protein powder and some healthy fats and you're cruising 'til lunchtime!

Add all the ingredients except the bee pollen to an upright blender and mix on high until the shake is thick and creamy, about 20 seconds.

Transfer to a large glass, top with the bee pollen if using, and serve immediately.

Serves 1

1 medium-size banana

2 cups baby spinach

1 celery stalk

1 tablespoon ground flaxseed

1 teaspoon spirulina powder

1 cup almond milk

1 teaspoon bee pollen for topping (optional)

Tips

Add a scoop of unflavored unsweetened protein powder to make it a complete meal.

You can top with hemp seeds instead of bee pollen.

For a dose of probiotics, add 2 heaping tablespoons of coconut yogurt.

If you would like your shake cold, add a handful of ice cubes.

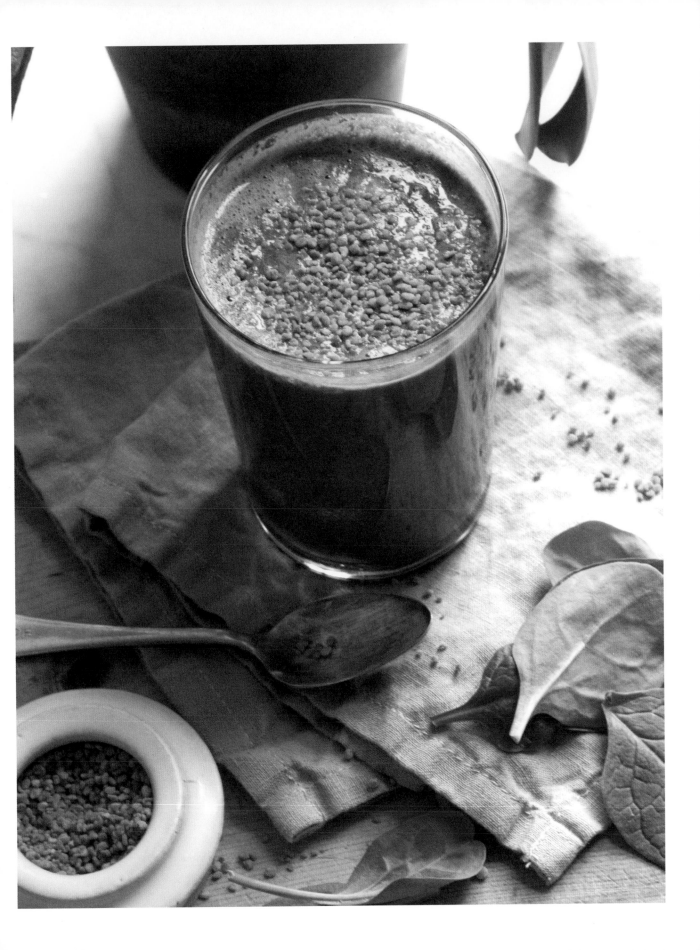

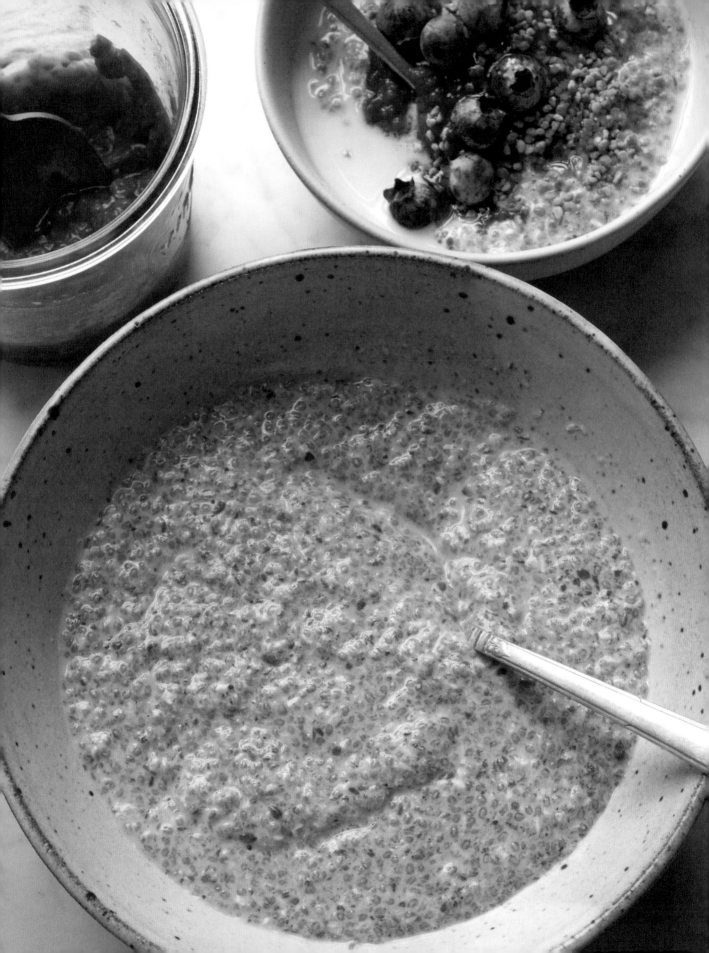

Creamy Overnight Seed Pudding

This rich, creamy pudding requires no cooking, is full of nutritious ingredients and fiber, is sugar-free, and comes together in five minutes. I like to make it at night and pop it in the fridge before I go to bed, knowing it will be waiting for me in the morning. It's great to have on hand if your schedule is busy. It's also nice to make when you have company and serve it family-style with fresh toppings on the side—just double or triple the recipe as needed to feed a crowd. Sometimes my husband drops a large spoonful of it into his smoothie, too, for a creamy boost.

Place all the ingredients in a glass bowl or food storage container and whisk until well combined.

Cover and place in the fridge for a minimum of 8 hours, or overnight.

When you're ready to eat, stir again and serve with toppings of your choice.

The pudding keeps well in the fridge for a week, covered.

Serves 2 to 4

¼ cup unsweetened shredded coconut

¼ cup ground flaxseed or flaxseed meal

¼ cup chia seeds

½ teaspoon ground cinnamon

1 tablespoon alcohol-free vanilla extract

2 cups almond milk

Toppings: berries, bee pollen, yogurt, compote, or honey

Swap It
Substitute any plant or dairy milk of your choice for the almond milk.

Tip
For a warm porridge, you can also heat it up gently on the stove with a splash of extra milk.

Grain-Free Granola

I'm a devoted label-reader. Besides perusing the produce isle at the market, I can mostly be found reading labels in search of products with the purest and cleanest ingredients. I'm looking for pantry items that aren't loaded with sugar, salt, pesticides, preservatives, hormones, antibiotics, industrial seed oils, or my favorite, "natural flavors." The rule of thumb I use is that most of my food should look a lot like how it looked when it came out of the ground, off the tree, from the farm, or out of the water. When I can't find what I'm looking for, my next attempt is to try to make it from scratch. Granola is a great example; when it's store-bought, it's one of those products that can be loaded with sugar and seed oils, but it's *very* easy to make at home. This low-carb, grain-free, gluten-free, nutrient-dense granola is full of good fats, fiber, protein, vitamins, and minerals and only has 1 tablespoon of maple syrup for a touch of sweetness. Warm scents of vanilla and cinnamon will fill your kitchen as it roasts. You can serve it over yogurt or ice cream, or just simply eat it with cold milk and honey. I leave a jar of it on the countertop, and family members scoop out handfuls to snack on as well.

Makes 5 cups

¼ cup coconut oil

1 tablespoon maple syrup

1 tablespoon alcohol-free vanilla extract

1 cup raw slivered almonds

1 cup raw walnut halves

1 cup raw pumpkin seeds

1 cup raw sunflower seeds

¼ cup almond flour

1 teaspoon ground cinnamon

Generous pinch of sea salt

Tip
Store for 2 weeks in the pantry or up to a month in the fridge.

Preheat the oven to 325°F, and line a large baking sheet with parchment paper.

In a small saucepan, melt the coconut oil and add the maple syrup and vanilla extract.

In a large bowl, combine and mix all the nuts and seeds.

Pour the wet ingredients over the nut-and-seed mixture, and stir everything together using a rubber spatula, making sure to coat it well. Add the almond flour, cinnamon, and salt and stir again.

Spread the mixture out evenly over the prepared baking sheet and roast for 10 to 13 minutes, until toasted and fragrant. Keep an eye on it to make sure it does not burn.

Remove the granola from the oven, and allow it to cool completely before transferring it to a few airtight glass containers or mason jars.

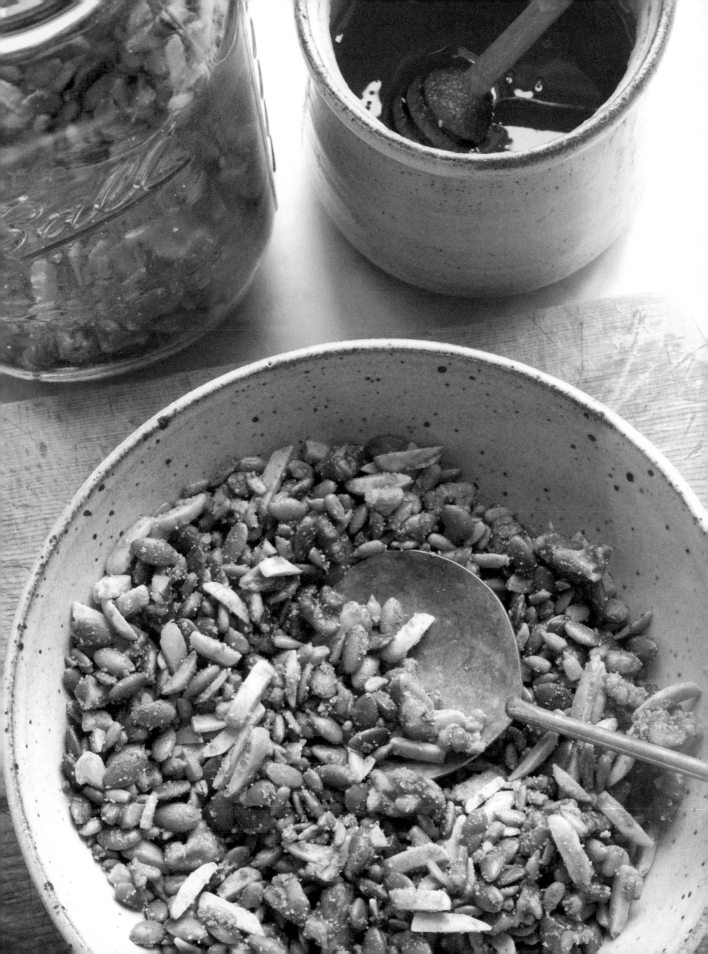

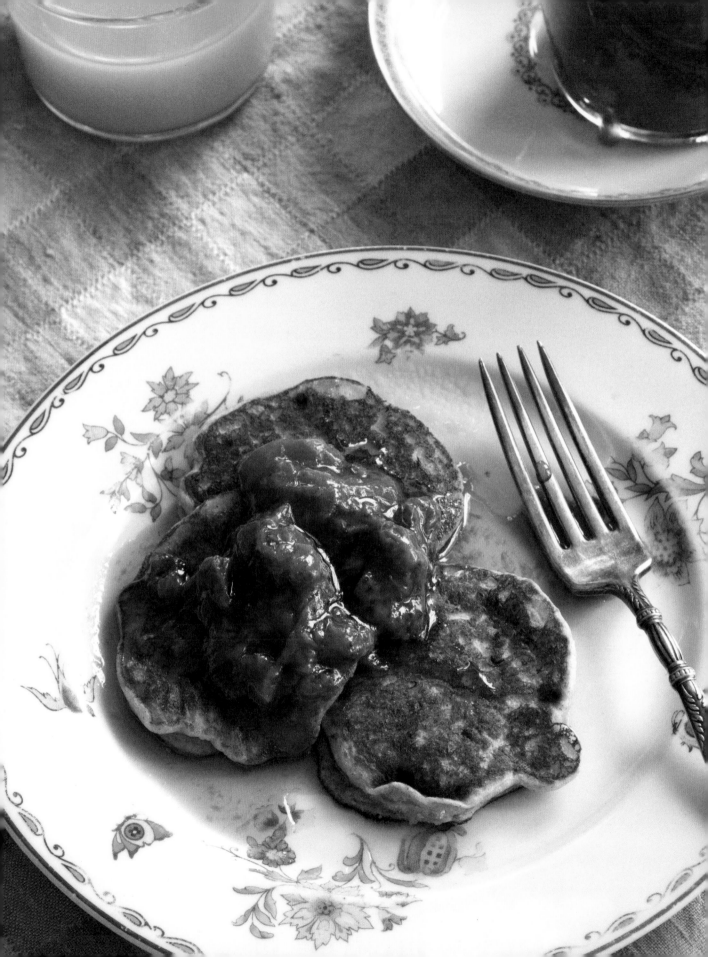

Fluffy Silver Dollar Pancakes

I grew up eating silver dollar pancakes with my dad at the Silver Star diner in New York City. When you're a kid, ordering the classic mini pancakes makes you feel like you've hit the jackpot because you get 10 times as many on your plate.

We have always taken pancakes very seriously in our house, but working with alternative ingredients can be tricky, especially when you're trying to get familiar textures. Our family's current favorite is grain-free, egg-free, and dairy-free. I've tested these a gazillion times, and discovered that this batter behaves best in a smaller format that reminds me of my old favorite silver dollars! They are fluffy, delicious, and kid-approved. Slather them in fruit compote and a touch of maple syrup. Heaven.

In a large mixing bowl, whisk the dry ingredients together until blended. In a medium bowl, mash the banana until almost smooth, then add all the other wet ingredients and whisk to blend. Add the wet ingredients to the dry ingredients and whisk until well combined. The batter should be thick.

Heat a large nonstick skillet over medium-low. Lightly grease the pan with oil and drop a few pancakes in, 1 heaping tablespoon of batter at a time. Don't overcrowd the pan. Cook for about a minute or so, or until golden brown on the underside. (You can gently lift the corner of a pancake with a rubber spatula to check before flipping.) Flip and finish cooking for another 1 to 2 minutes, or until browned on the second side; then transfer to a serving dish and cover with a dish towel to keep warm. Repeat with the remaining batter.

You can transfer the batter to an airtight container and store in the fridge for 3 days.

Makes about 20 (2½-inch) pancakes

1 cup blanched almond flour

½ cup arrowroot flour

¼ cup coconut flour

2 teaspoons aluminum-free baking powder

½ teaspoon kosher sea salt

½ teaspoon ground cinnamon

¾ cup mashed banana (from 2 to 3 bananas)

1½ cups almond milk

2 tablespoons avocado oil, plus more for the skillet

1 tablespoon alcohol-free vanilla extract

1 tablespoon apple cider vinegar

Tips

To reheat the pancakes, transfer them to an oven-safe dish and warm at 250°F for 10 to 15 minutes, or until heated through. Serve with Vanilla Berry Compote (page 32) or really go for it and add fresh fruit and maple syrup.

You could also add ¼ cup blueberries or chocolate chips to the batter.

Wild Blueberry Muffins

With barely six grams of sugar each, these muffins are a lovely warm and nourishing treat in the morning if you're looking for something to grab and go. They are grain-free and full of healthy fats. Perfectly sweet and bright thanks to a squeeze of citrus juice, they bake up with a slightly crunchy exterior and tender crumb. For extra fun, slice them in half and toast them cut side down in a pan with a little ghee, New York City deli–style, then slather with jam or Vanilla Berry Compote (page 32).

Preheat the oven to 350°F, and line a 12-cup muffin tin with paper baking cups.

In a medium bowl, whisk together the ground flaxseed, psyllium husks, and lemon zest. Then mix in all the wet ingredients and set aside.

In a large bowl, whisk together all the dry ingredients (through salt). Add the wet ingredients to the dry ingredients and mix with a rubber spatula. (The batter will be thick.) Fold in the blueberries.

Using an ice-cream scoop or measuring cup, drop about ¼ cup of batter into each baking cup. Bake for 30 to 35 minutes, or until golden brown and a toothpick or fork inserted in the center of a muffin comes out clean.

Remove from the oven and allow to cool for 10 minutes in the pan, then transfer to a wire rack to cool completely.

Serve immediately, or store in an airtight container at room temperature for up to 3 days or in the fridge for 1 week. Bring back to room temperature or toast before serving.

Makes about 12 muffins

2 tablespoons ground flaxseed or flaxseed meal

3 tablespoons whole psyllium husks

1 tablespoon lemon zest

¾ cup almond milk

½ cup avocado oil

⅓ cup maple syrup

1 tablespoon alcohol-free vanilla extract

2 tablespoons fresh lemon juice

2 cups superfine blanched almond flour

¼ cup coconut flour

¼ cup arrowroot flour

¼ cup unsweetened shredded dried coconut

2 teaspoons baking powder

¼ teaspoon kosher sea salt

1 cup frozen wild blueberries

Swap It
You can use orange zest and juice instead of lemon if you prefer.

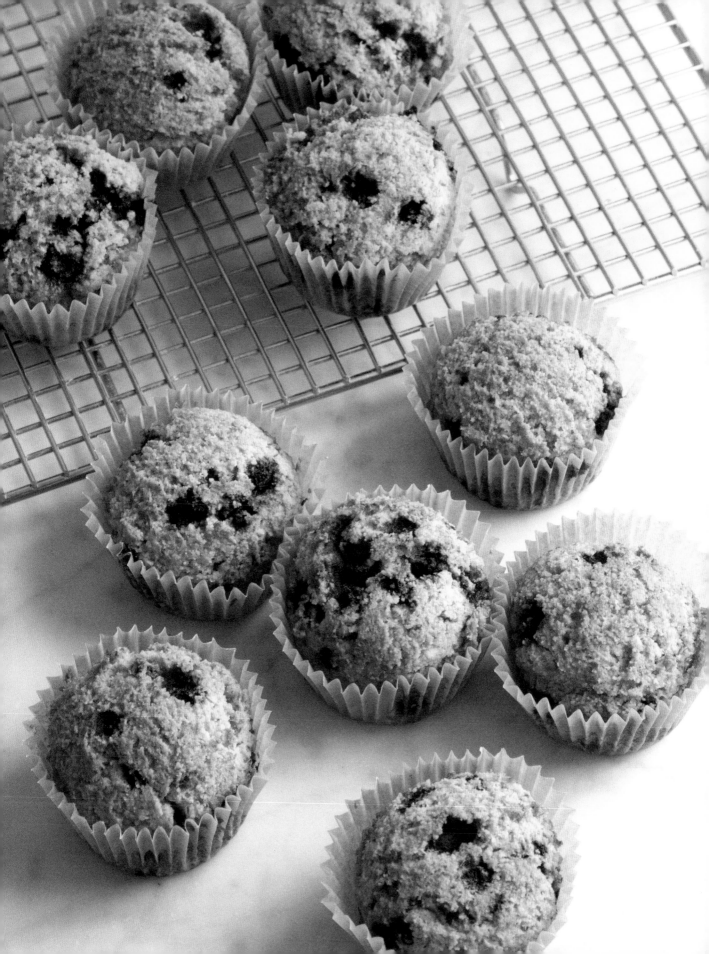

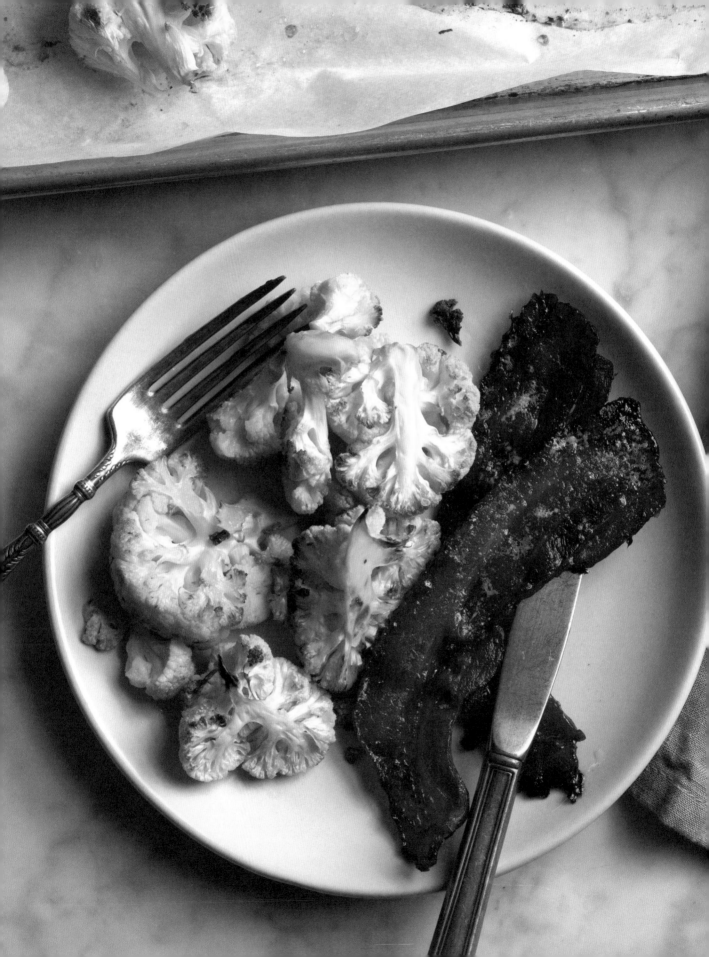

Maple Bacon + Veg

Oh, the joy of cooking bacon on a sheet pan! When you use this method, you won't get smoked out of your kitchen or have to deal with a greasy, messy cleanup. In this egg-free take on a bacon-and-egg breakfast, everything crisps up together beautifully in one pan in the oven, making this super easy and great for serving company. I like thick-cut bacon because it has more fat and protein, which means more flavor and chew when caramelized with the maple syrup. I'm allergic to eggs, but I love the familiar play on visuals here: the cauliflower really does become an excellent scrambled egg stand-in. I've added a touch of maple syrup to the bacon to amp up the breakfast vibes, but you could skip that if you're avoiding sugar.

Preheat the oven to 400°F, and line a large baking sheet with parchment paper.

Lay individual pieces of bacon out together, side by side, on one end of the pan. Place the cauliflower on the other end of the pan, drizzle with the olive oil, sprinkle with salt, and toss by hand to mix well. Spread the cauliflower out evenly.

Roast for 20 minutes, then place the pan on the stove top. Flip each piece of bacon and drizzle with the maple syrup. Place the sheet pan back in the oven and continue roasting for another 15 to 20 minutes, until the bacon is deeply browned and crisp.

Remove from the oven and serve straight from the pan or transfer to a serving dish.

Serves 2 to 4

1 (8-ounce) package thick-cut uncured bacon

1 head of cauliflower (1 to 1½ pounds), chopped into 2-inch pieces

3 tablespoons extra-virgin olive oil

¾ teaspoon kosher sea salt

1 tablespoon maple syrup

Tip
You can add another tablespoon of maple syrup if you prefer your bacon extra sweet. You can also toss the cauliflower with ½ teaspoon of ground turmeric, ground paprika, or ground cumin for extra flavor.

Beans, Greens + Broken Eggs

I like a well-rounded savory and filling breakfast that doesn't require a lot of prep time. If you happen to have a Big Batch of Beans (page 40) lying around, this dish will come together quickly. If not, you can easily pop open a can of beans instead. The key here is cooking the eggs just right. Making them over easy allows for fully cooked whites with a soft yolk that breaks open easily, allowing the rich insides to spill down over the beans and greens. It's sort of a self-saucing situation.

Heat a large nonstick skillet over medium. Add the olive oil and garlic and sauté for just 1 minute, until fragrant, then add the greens and salt. Using tongs, toss the greens around until they have shrunken and softened, about 3 minutes for softer greens like spinach, or up to 5 minutes for tougher greens like rainbow chard and mustard greens. Then transfer them to a plate.

Add the ghee to the pan. When it has melted, crack the eggs into the pan with even spacing. Season with salt and pepper if you wish. Cook each egg until there is about a ½ inch of unset white surrounding each yolk. Using a spatula, carefully flip the eggs, making sure to separate them gently if the whites have run into each other. Once the eggs are flipped, turn the heat off and let them sit in the pan for a minute.

To plate up, add half the beans to each of two wide bowls, then place half the cooked greens over each pile of beans. Set an over-easy egg on top of each and season with more salt and pepper and a drizzle of olive oil. Serve immediately, breaking the eggs as you dig in.

Serves 2

1 tablespoon extra-virgin olive oil, plus more for serving

1 clove garlic, minced

1 bunch (about 6 ounces) of leafy greens (such as rainbow chard, mustard greens, or spinach), ends trimmed and roughly chopped

½ teaspoon kosher sea salt, plus more for seasoning

2 tablespoons ghee

2 large eggs

Freshly ground black pepper (optional)

1½ cups cooked beans, warmed (from Big Batch of Beans, page 40, or canned beans)

Sauce It
You can top the eggs with a few spoonfuls of Cherry Tomato Confit (page 18) or House Pesto (page 10).

Tip
You can add a serving of Carnitas (page 185) or Citrus-Cured Lox (page 145) for more protein.

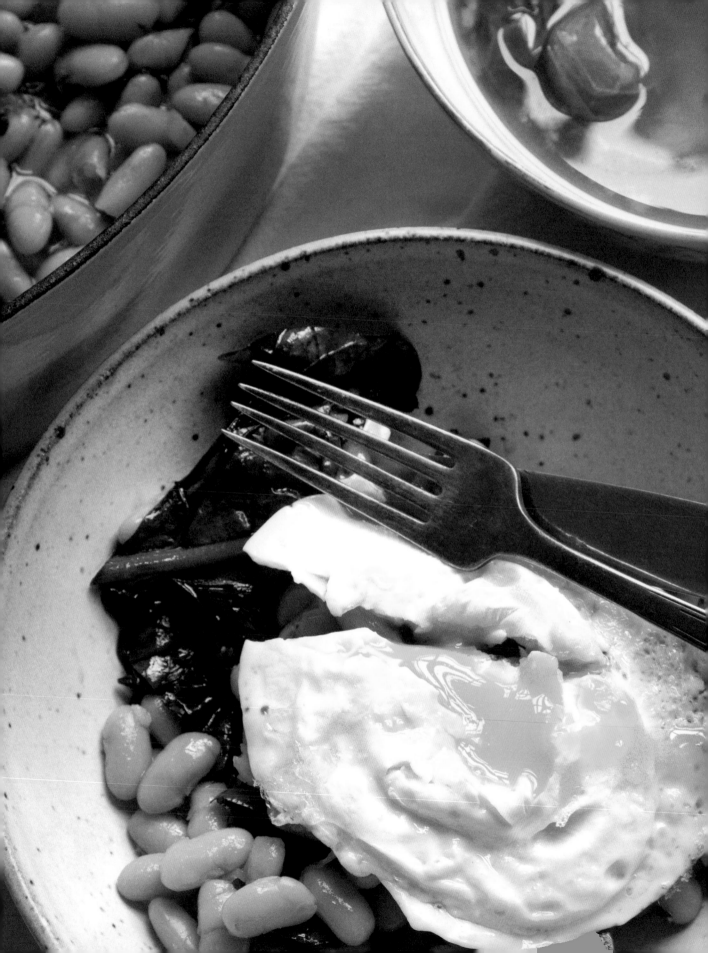

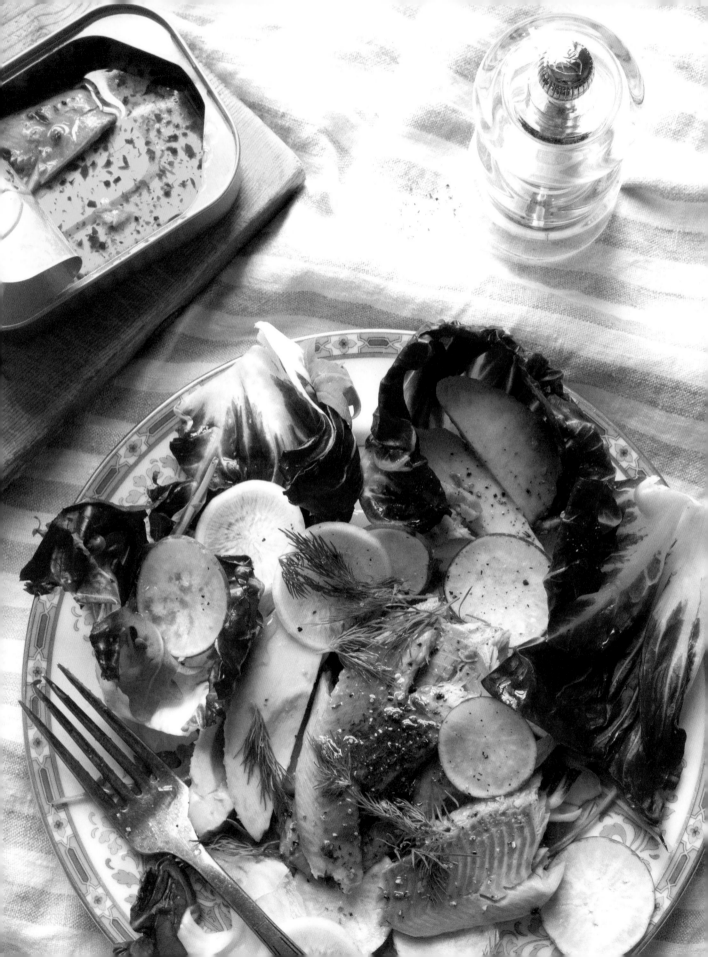

Tinned Fish Breakfast Salad

Sardines are a must-have pantry staple in our house. Believe it or not, this is my go-to breakfast most days of the week. Hear me out. I realize tinned fish is not for everyone, but I grew up on the stuff and find it to be the perfect quick fix for flavor and nutrition. Bright peppery arugula or crisp radicchio, crunchy vegetables, creamy avocado, fresh herbs, and lemon juice balance out the rich oily fish. I also love sardines, trout, and mackerel because they are full of protein, omega-3 fatty acids, vitamin D, and calcium. What's more, I can assemble this powerhouse breakfast plate in five minutes. If you are working on a health issue that requires you to be diligent, tinned seafood can be helpful when your food options are limited—I have been known to travel with sardines.

Arrange the arugula or the radicchio on a salad plate. Open the tinned fish and carefully lift the pieces out, placing them on the bed of greens. Set the tin aside; you'll use the oil later.

Layer the avocado and radish slices around the fish and top with the dill. Drizzle with the olive oil and 1 tablespoon of the olive oil from the tin. Squeeze the lemon juice over and sprinkle with salt.

Serves 1

2 cups fresh arugula or radicchio

1 (roughly 4-ounce) tin of fish (such as sardines, trout, mackerel, or shellfish) packed in olive oil

½ medium avocado, sliced

2 radishes, thinly sliced

¼ cup roughly chopped fresh dill

1 tablespoon extra-virgin olive oil

Juice of half a lemon

Pinch of kosher sea salt

Freshly ground black pepper (optional)

Swap It
You can substitute cured or leftover salmon or jarred wild tuna for the tinned fish. You can also swap out the arugula and use fresh spinach, mixed greens, or bitter lettuces instead, or try parsley or cilantro instead of dill.

Sauce It
Instead of using the fresh lemon juice and olive oil, try Marlit's Vinaigrette (page 8).

Tip
You can also pile this whole plate onto a thick slice of toast or serve it over a bowl of steaming rice.

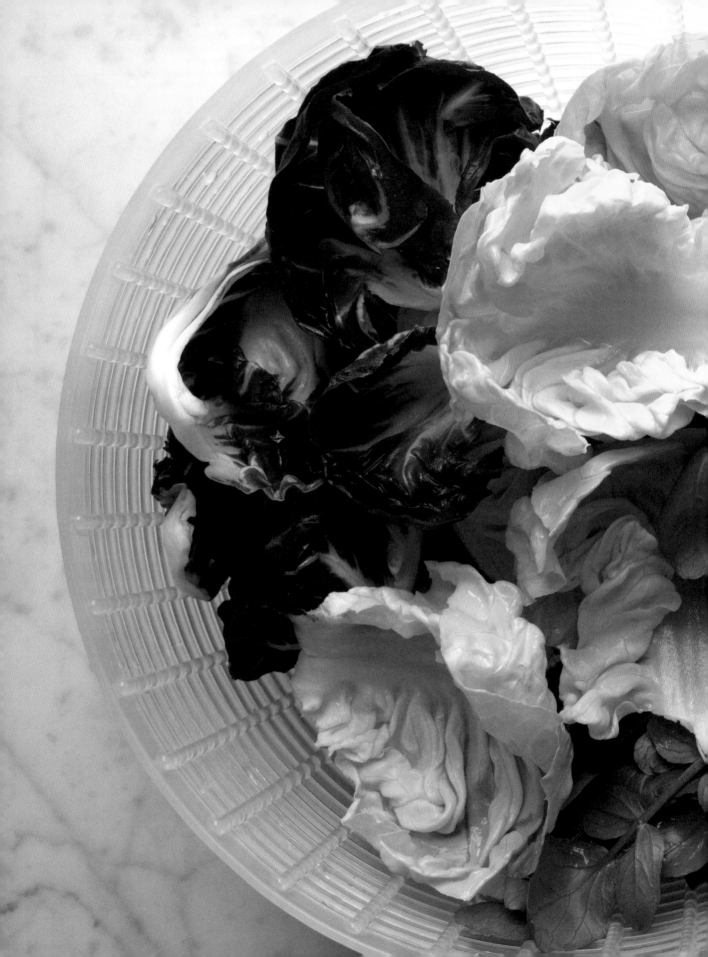

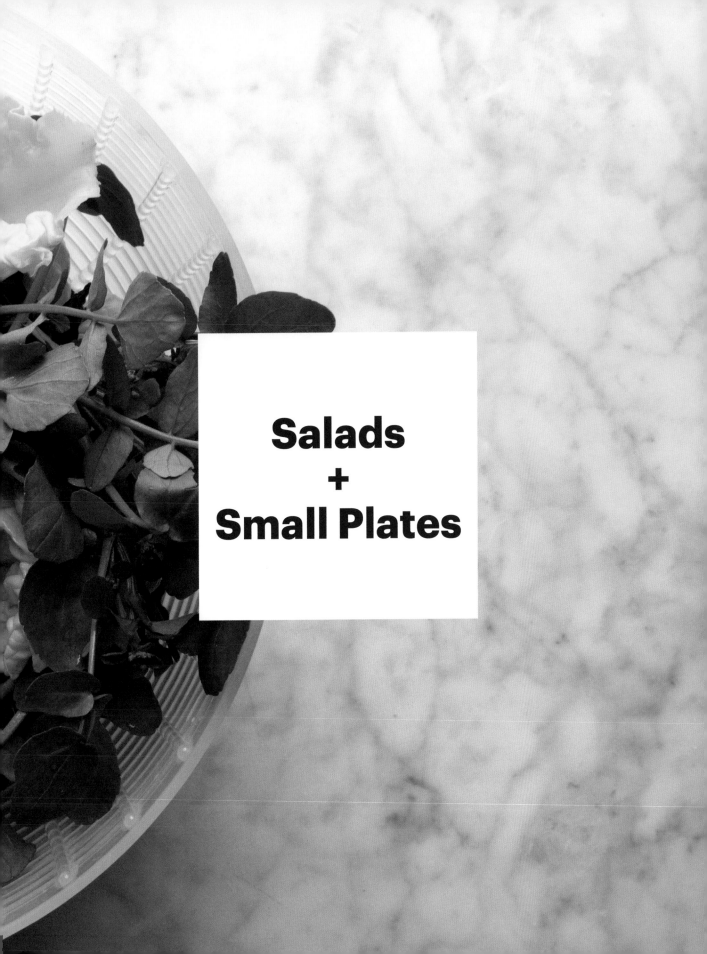

Salads
+
Small Plates

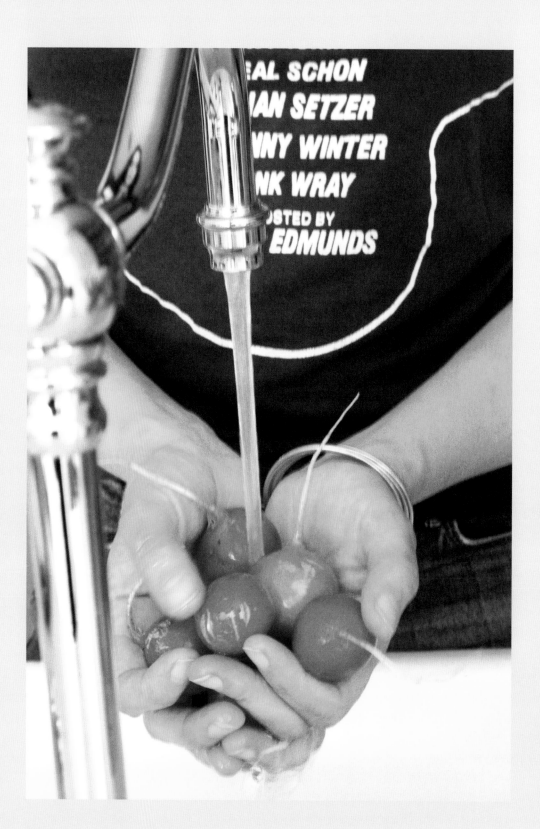

Food Ego

What we eat is a huge part of our identity. Our food represents our joys, love, family culture, memories, economic status, self-worth, emotional life, fears, travels, and more. There is a lot of information on our plates. When we change the food we eat, we are addressing much bigger issues in our lives, and we are communicating something new to the world and to our hearts. Making big changes to your eating habits is hard, and your family and friends might not understand at first.

When I discovered that my path to recovery was primarily through food, I was all in. I love to eat and I love to cook, so it made perfect sense to me: I knew I could learn new recipes, find new ingredients, and leave behind anything that didn't support my health to heal my body. *What a joy,* I thought. *I may not have to take drugs, and instead I can cook and eat my way back to vibrant health!* Nearly two decades later, I can proudly say that I'm the healthiest I've ever been (and medication-free) at almost 50 years old. I feel good, I have energy, I feel nourished, and I sleep well.

But there were plenty of challenges and setbacks along the way. My food identity suffered quite a bit in the beginning of my health journey, too. I discovered that I wanted to be seen as someone who loves food and has an exciting and adventurous palate, even though I was choosing a new way of eating that may have had a reputation for being less delicious. My food ego had been constructed around many foods that didn't love me back, and cutting those out felt like losing an important part of me. There were rumblings from friends and family; some people thought less of the kind of food I was eating and made jokes and sarcastic comments. I sometimes thought I'd have to choose between eating healthy and loving my food. But over time, I've realized I can have both worlds. I feed myself what my body needs, but I also eat exciting, stimulating, inspiring meals all the time. Have faith: you are not sentenced to a life of bland and boring food when you change your diet. In fact, feeling better tastes *so* good.

Butter Lettuce with Fresh Herbs, Toasted Maple Sunflower Seeds + Marlit's Vinaigrette

My grandmother Marlit was famous in our family for her salad and dressing. As a child, I used to stand at the foot of her kitchen island, helping her make this classic French salad of simple dressed greens. She would first soak leaves of butter lettuce in a big tub of cold water to help pull the dirt from them. They emerged tender and crisp, and we would carefully break them apart into large pieces and dry them in the salad spinner and then on dish cloths. Next, she would toss them gently in a bowl with a few spoonfuls of her vinaigrette. Here's my version; I've added some fresh herbs to the leaves and topped everything off with sweet, tiny sunflower seeds to add some crunch.

Serves 2

2 heads of butter, Boston, or Bibb lettuce (5 to 7 ounces each)

Leaves from 2 large stems of tarragon

Small handful of fresh dill, torn or roughly chopped

Marlit's Vinaigrette (page 8)

¼ cup Toasted Maple Sunflower Seeds (page 35)

Fill up the bowl of a salad spinner and inner basket with cold water and add a few handfuls of ice cubes. Gently pull apart the first head of lettuce, discarding any damaged leaves, and drop the good ones into the bowl. Carefully swirl the leaves around in the ice water and let them sit for a few minutes while you prepare the dressing. This will help the lettuce crisp up.

Drain and spin the lettuce dry, then transfer to a large salad bowl and repeat with the second head of lettuce until everything is crisp, clean, and dry. At this point, you can cover the bowl with plastic wrap and store it in the fridge for up to 4 hours, if you'd like to make this in advance.

When you are ready to assemble the salad, wash your hands. Add the torn herbs to the lettuce bowl, then drizzle with ¼ cup of the salad dressing to start and toss gently by hand, making sure to coat all the leaves. Taste and add more dressing to your liking. Stack the leaves onto plates, sprinkle with the toasted sunflower seeds, and serve immediately.

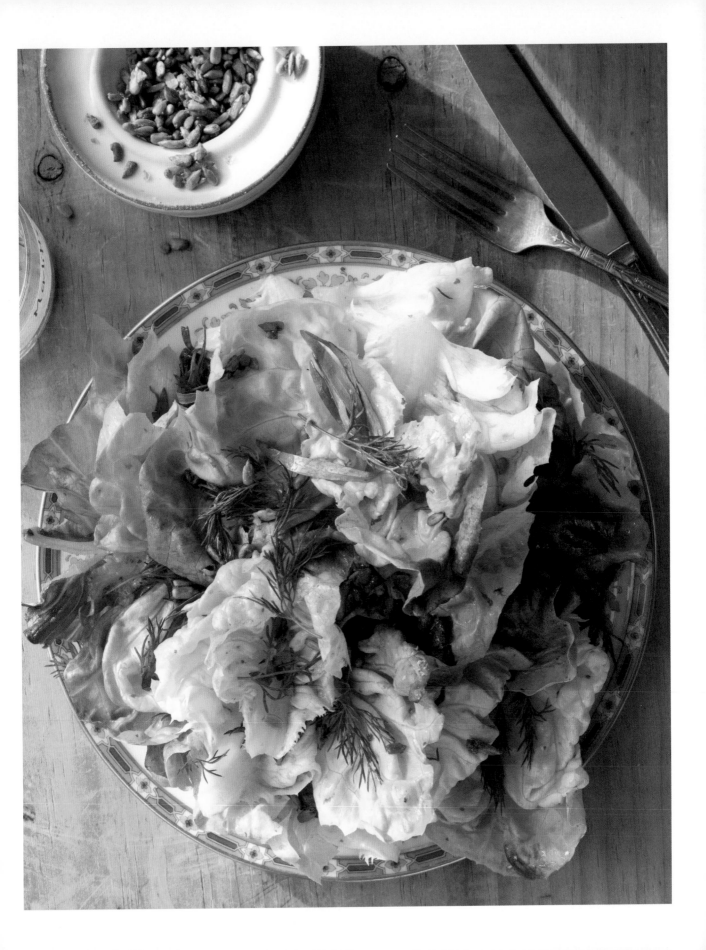

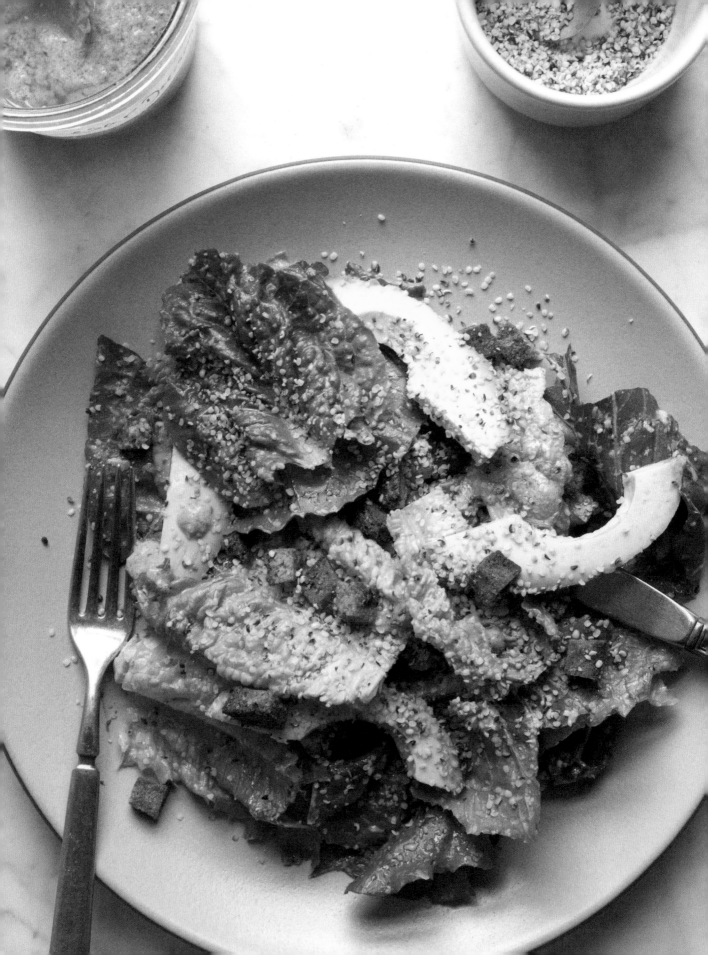

Caesar Salad with Avocado, Croutons + Hemp Seeds

This version of one of my favorite salads is gluten- and dairy-free, and topped with Cheesy Garlic Croutons (page 12) made from the Grain-Free Vegan Boule (page 201). I promise you that if you share this dish with people who don't have food allergies, they won't notice that they're missing anything. It has all the important elements of a classic Caesar, with lots of crunch and a rich, punchy dressing made with anchovies. I've topped it all off with avocados and hemp seeds to boost nutrition.

Place the lettuce in a large salad bowl and add the dressing. Toss together, add the croutons, and toss again.

To plate up, divide the salad among plates and top each one with a few slices of avocado and a sprinkle of about 1 tablespoon of hemp seeds. Serve with extra dressing and croutons on the side.

Serves 6

2 heads of romaine lettuce (about 10 ounces each), washed and torn into bite-size pieces

½ cup Caesar Dressing (page 9), plus more if needed

1 cup Cheesy Garlic Croutons (page 12), plus more if needed

2 medium avocados (about 7 ounces each), sliced for serving

Hemp seeds, for serving

Tuscan Kale Salad with Pomegranate, Pine Nuts + Currants

I love to serve this at Thanksgiving and other holidays to add a fresh element to sometimes-heavy holiday menus. All the components of this salad come together beautifully. It's super easy to make because the dressing is simply a drizzle of olive oil, freshly squeezed orange juice, and balsamic vinegar. One important thing to note here: Massage the kale. Don't skip this step. The process helps break down the tough fibers in this sturdy leafy green, making it much easier to chew. This hearty salad also keeps well in the fridge after it's been dressed, so enjoy it for a few days if you have leftovers—or in the case of a holiday meal, make it a few days ahead.

In a large salad bowl, combine the kale with the olive oil and the salt and massage for 3 to 5 minutes, or until it has softened and reduced in size a little.

Add the fresh orange zest and juice and continue to massage a little more, adding extra olive oil if necessary, 1 teaspoon at a time, until the leaves are tender and glossy.

Add the remaining ingredients and toss a final time to make sure everything is coated in the dressing and mixed well. Taste and adjust seasoning if necessary.

Serve immediately, or store in an airtight container in the fridge for up to 3 days.

Serves 4 to 6

- 2 heads of Tuscan kale (about 10 ounces each), tough ribs removed, torn into 2-inch pieces
- 3 tablespoons extra-virgin olive oil, plus more if needed
- ½ teaspoon kosher sea salt
- 1 teaspoon orange zest
- 3 tablespoons freshly squeezed orange juice (from half a juicy orange)
- 2 tablespoons syrupy balsamic vinegar
- ¼ cup thinly sliced red onion
- ¼ cup dried currants
- ¼ cup pomegranate seeds
- ¼ cup toasted pine nuts (see Tip on page 25)
- Freshly ground black pepper

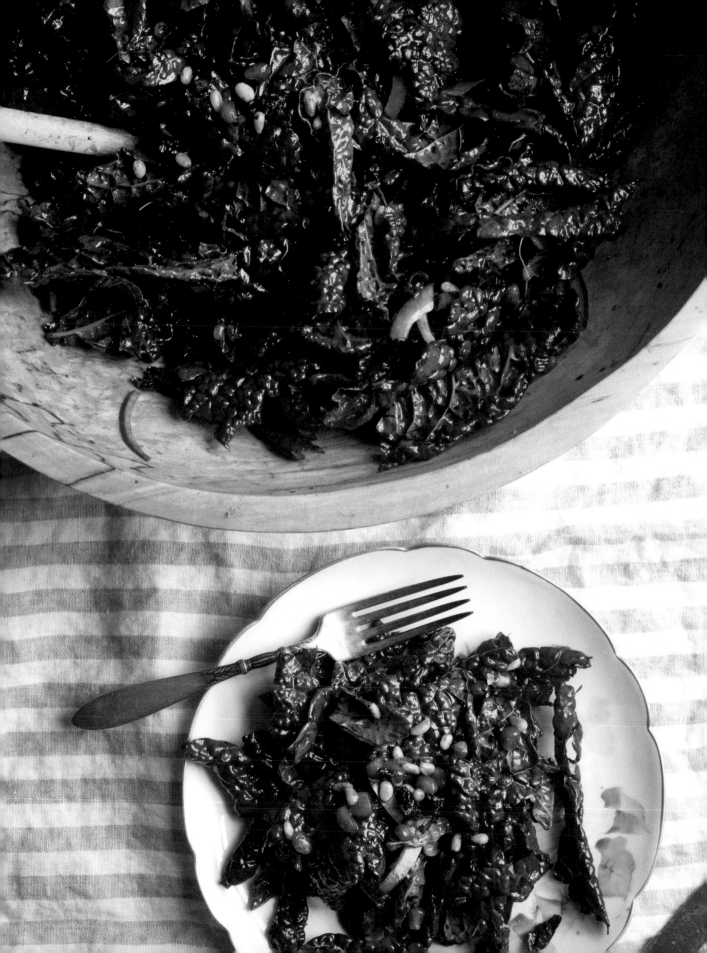

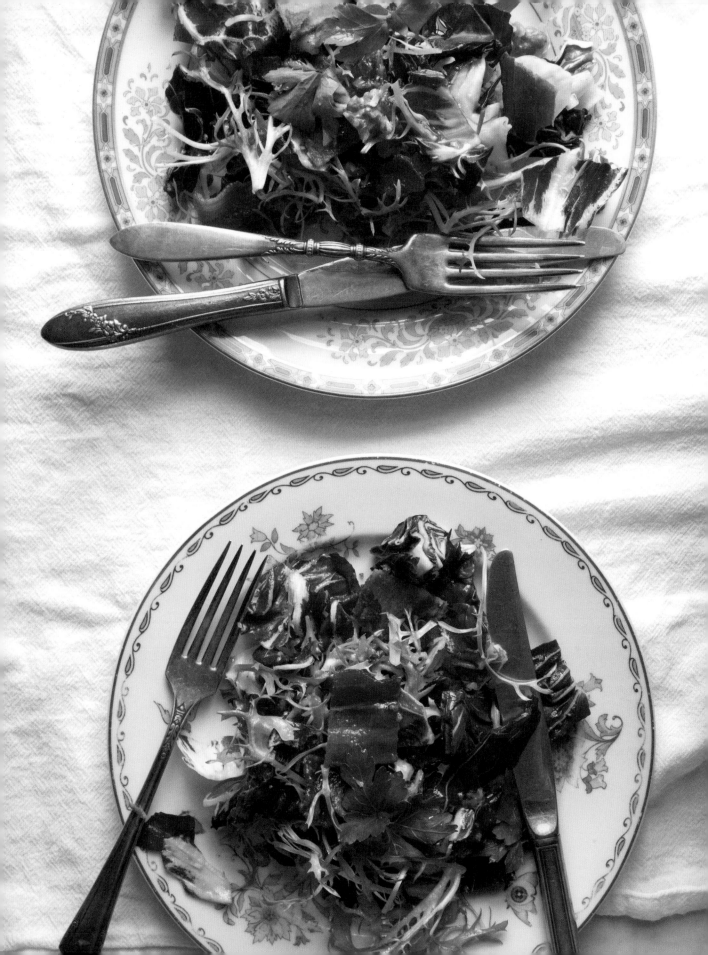

Chicory Chop Salad

Bitter chicory lettuces are bold and call for assertive flavors to balance out their strong characteristics. I also love them because they are nutrient-dense and support gut health. They are full of prebiotic material that helps feed the good bacteria in your gut. An old friend turned me onto the brilliance of a chopped salad, where everything is cut into same-size pieces, making it easy to scoop up all the components together in every bite! I think this chicory chop is a fun and more dynamic take on a classic chopped salad and pairs perfectly with the Whole-Lemon Anchovy Dressing (page 9).

Preheat the oven to 375°F.

Lay the bacon slices out side by side on a baking sheet lined with parchment paper and roast for 15 to 20 minutes, until crispy.

Remove from the oven and let cool for 10 minutes; then transfer the bacon to a paper towel–lined plate to drain before roughly chopping. Roast the walnuts on a small baking sheet lined with parchment paper for about 8 minutes, until golden, then let cool slightly and roughly chop. Allow to cool completely.

In a large salad bowl, combine the radicchio, frisée, onion, and parsley and gently toss together by hand. Add the bacon and walnuts, and drizzle with about ¼ cup of the dressing to start. Toss again, taste, and add more dressing as necessary. Season with salt and pepper. Serve immediately.

Serves 2 to 3 as a meal, or 4 to 6 as a side

1 (8-ounce) package organic uncured bacon (such as from Applegate Sunday)

⅓ cup walnuts

1 large head of radicchio (about 12 ounces), roughly chopped into bite-size pieces

½ head of frisée or escarole (about 4 ounces), chopped into bite-size pieces

¼ cup finely chopped red onion

½ cup roughly chopped fresh flat-leaf parsley

Whole-Lemon Anchovy Dressing (page 9)

Kosher sea salt

Freshly ground black pepper

Tips

To bulk up this salad as a main course, you can add chopped avocado, hard-boiled eggs, pitted green olives, or the Cheesy Garlic Croutons (page 12).

For a vegan version, leave out the bacon and use an anchovy-free dressing.

Heirloom Tomato Salad

This recipe is dedicated to all the nightshade lovers and tolerators out there. I see you. There are two important things to note here: First, salting the tomatoes in advance and letting them sit for 15 to 20 minutes will transform the fruit by drawing out its natural juices and intensifying its flavors. Second, try to find the best in-season heirloom tomatoes possible. Maybe you have a vegetable garden, a good friend with a vegetable garden, or a local farmers' market. Go out of your way to seek the juiciest, ripest fruit you can. If you do all of this, you could serve the tomatoes as is with a drizzle of olive oil. However, if you are looking to add something more, I suggest Marlit's Vinaigrette (page 8).

Place the tomatoes in a deep serving platter, gently toss them with the salt, and let rest for 15 to 20 minutes to develop flavor and draw out juices.

When ready to serve, add fresh pepper and drizzle with olive oil. If you are using the dressing, you can drizzle some over the olive oil as well, or serve it on the side for each person to apply. Top with crumbled bacon and fresh herbs if desired.

Serves 4 to 6

2 pounds heirloom tomatoes, sliced into thick slabs or wedges

½ teaspoon kosher sea salt

Freshly ground black pepper

3 tablespoons extra-virgin olive oil

¼ cup Marlit's Vinaigrette (optional), plus more as needed

2 to 3 pieces bacon, cooked and crumbled (optional)

1 to 2 tablespoons chopped fresh herbs, such as parsley, dill, or thyme (optional)

Tip
Serve on a warm summer night with grilled steak or for lunch spooned over some garlic toast made from the Grain-Free Vegan Boule (page 201).

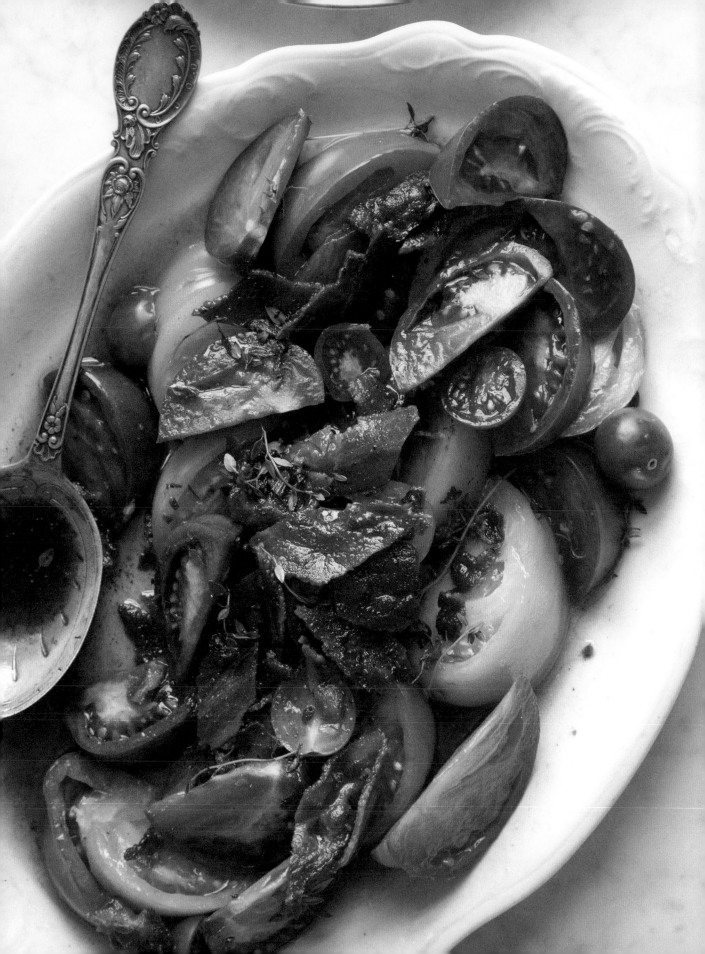

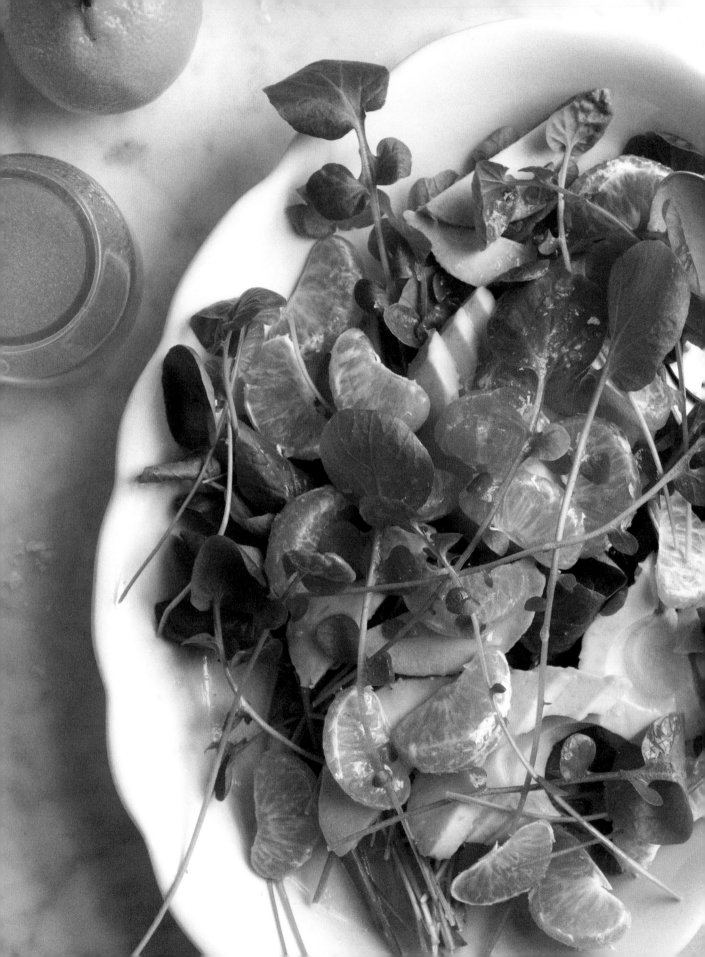

Mandarin, Avocado + Watercress Salad

This salad is sunshine on a plate, a welcome vision during the winter months, when citrus is in season and the days are short. Alice Waters put this combo on the map for me. The sweet-and-juicy tanginess of citrus fruit coupled with luscious avocado and peppery greens are a perfect ensemble.

In a small bowl, whisk together the mandarin juice, vinegar, oil, and salt.

Make a bed with the watercress leaves on a medium serving dish. Arrange avocado slices over the greens and add the mandarin segments. Drizzle the dressing over the salad and season with sea salt and fresh black pepper if using. Toss gently and serve immediately.

Serves 2

2 tablespoons freshly squeezed mandarin juice

2 teaspoons Champagne vinegar

2 tablespoons extra-virgin olive oil

⅛ teaspoon kosher sea salt, plus more for seasoning

1 bunch of watercress (about 2 ounces)

1 Hass avocado, pit removed and thinly sliced

3 mandarins, peeled, segments separated

Freshly cracked pepper (optional)

Swap It
You can substitute other citrus sections, like blood orange or grapefruit, for the mandarins. You can also substitute arugula for the watercress if you prefer.

Tip
Add 8 ounces of grilled chicken or salmon to make it more of a main course.

Curried Wild Tuna Salad

This is a quick go-to lunch recipe that comes together fast and is bursting with sweet-and-savory flavors and textures. It's bright, crunchy, and tart. I prefer yogurt here to mayonnaise for an added dose of midday probiotics. You can serve this on toast for a sandwich or simply snack on it plated with crisp vegetables and seed crackers. I like to start off with jarred wild tuna packed in olive oil for extra-healthy luscious fats that create a rich base for the rest of these fresh ingredients. Be mindful that tuna is higher in mercury than most other fish and should be eaten in moderation.

In a medium bowl, combine all the ingredients and fold together using a large spoon until everything is well mixed. Serve immediately, or transfer to an airtight container and store in the fridge for up to 3 days.

Serves 4

2 (6-ounce) jars wild tuna in olive oil

½ small red onion, finely chopped (about ⅓ cup)

½ cup finely chopped celery (from 1 large stalk)

1 tablespoon country-style Dijon mustard

1 teaspoon lemon zest plus 1 tablespoon fresh lemon juice (from 1 lemon)

¼ cup unsweetened, plain Greek-style coconut yogurt (such as Cocojune Pure Coconut)

3 tablespoons finely chopped fresh dill

1½ teaspoons curry powder

½ Honeycrisp apple, finely chopped (about ⅔ cup)

¼ teaspoon kosher sea salt

Swap It

Substitute raisins or halved red grapes for the apple.

To make this vegan, substitute 1 can of drained and rinsed chickpeas for the tuna. Simply mash the beans roughly with a fork and mix with all the ingredients above, adding 2 to 4 tablespoons of extra-virgin olive oil as needed.

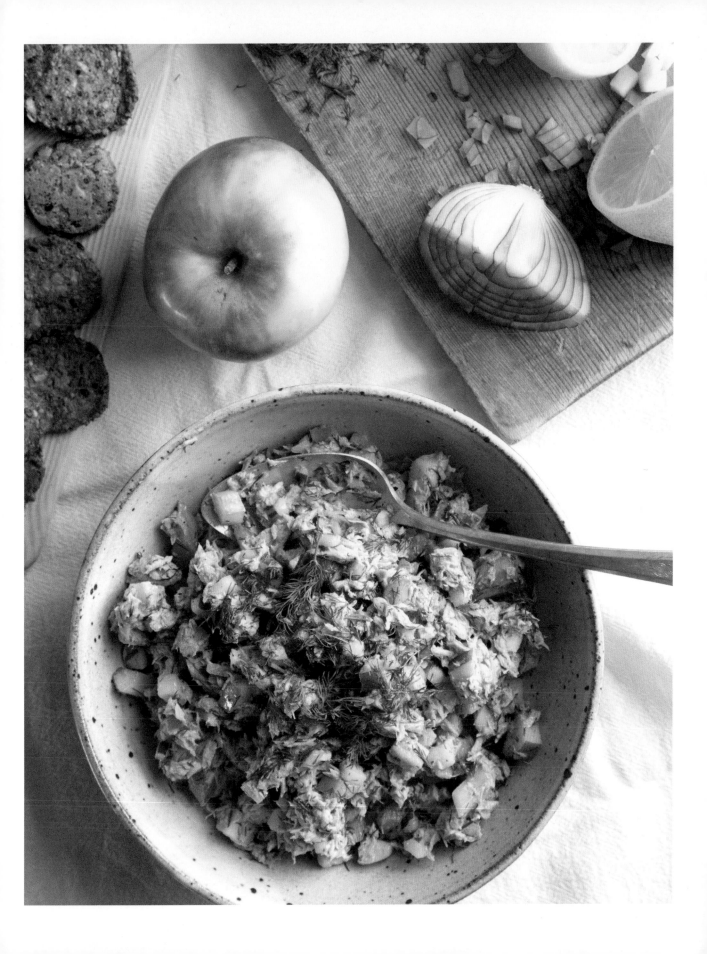

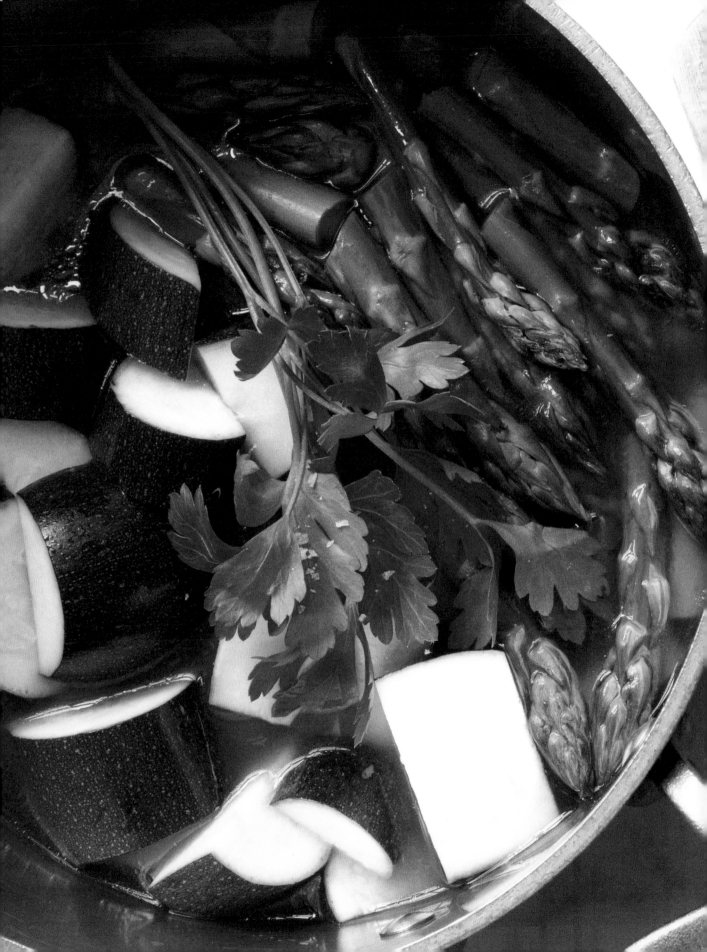

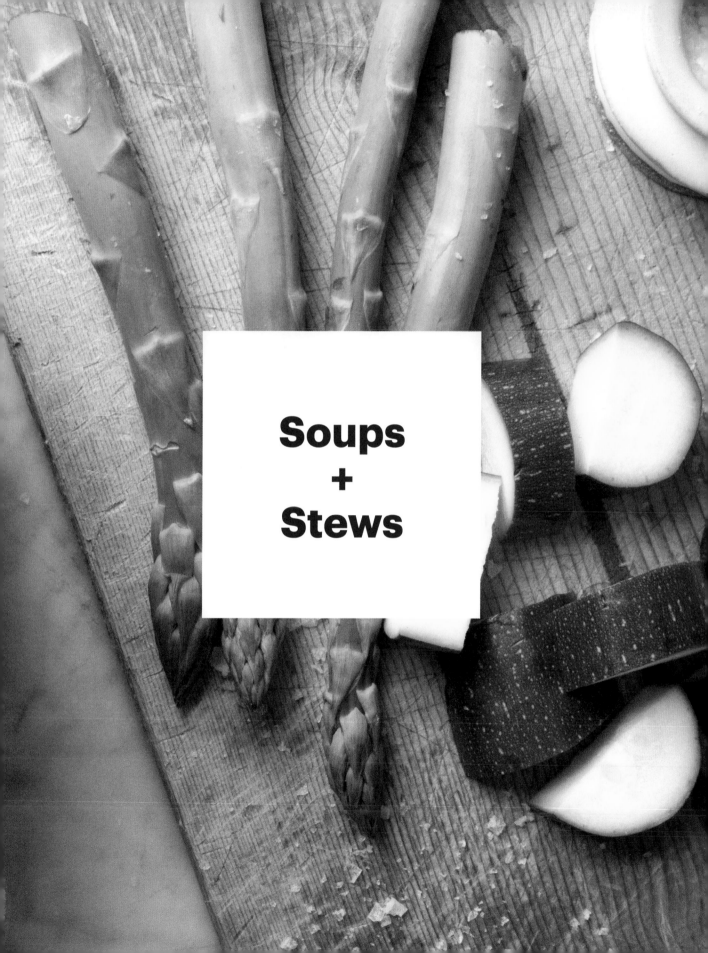

Soups
+
Stews

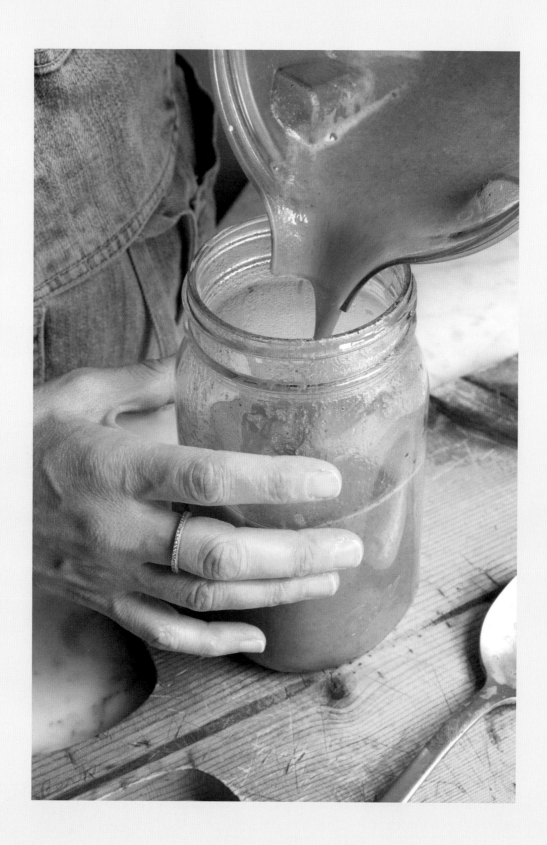

Food Is Medicine

When I was first diagnosed with Hashimoto's disease, an autoimmune disorder that affects the thyroid gland, my doctor at the time gave me medication and told me that I was lucky to have an illness that could be easily medicated for the rest of my life. *The rest of my life?!* I thought. *Oh no, there must be another way.* His words lit a fire in my belly. I set out to understand the root cause of my condition, and almost two decades later, I still haven't looked back. I learned that it is sometimes possible to reverse autoimmune disease and heal naturally with the help of a good doctor, support from your family and friends, and a dedicated nutrition and lifestyle plan—particularly one that focuses on healing the gut. I have experienced the undeniable power of nutrition.

It is so very important that you know how powerful your food is and the impact it has on your health. Getting sick can be painful and confusing, but above all, it is an invitation from your body. Your body is communicating to you all the time. Listening to the signals your body is sending is one of the first steps toward recovery. Finding a good doctor is crucial, but it is only part of the work. Nobody knows your body better than you. There is so much you can do at home in your kitchen to help heal and rebalance your system, and the good news is that it can complement whatever plan you and your doctor decide is best for you.

Cooking for yourself is empowering because it gives you the opportunity to control exactly what goes into your body. If you're not used to preparing your own meals regularly, or you don't have time to cook during the week, try making a big pot of soup on the weekend that can carry you through the first few days of the week. Rotisserie Chicken Soup (page 91), Red Lentil Mulligatawny Soup (page 95), or Bone Broth Vegetable Purée (page 88) can provide lots of nourishment, and they are all so easy to prepare and reheat. If you work from home, you may find that cooking dinner in the morning when you have more energy is a more sustainable way to get home-cooked meals on the table. Either way, as you lean into taking care of yourself, you will discover (as I did) that food is medicine.

Bone Broth Vegetable Purée

Every meal I make is designed to support my health in some way. Blending together the medicinal properties of bone broth with phyto-nutrients and vegetable fiber makes this a complete and powerful meal that's super easy to digest. I especially like to have this on hand during the winter months, when rich meals are abundant and I need clean and calming nourishment in between holiday dinners and gatherings to help me stay balanced. You can experiment with any vegetables you like to formulate your own blends. This is the broccoli version, but you can substitute 3 cups of almost any vegetable for the broccoli, adjusting the cooking times until the vegetable is tender. My favorites are broccoli, zucchini, spinach, asparagus, carrots, and butternut squash.

Heat a medium pot over medium for about 3 minutes. Add the olive oil, the onions, and ½ teaspoon of the salt and stir together. Reduce heat to medium-low and cook until the onions are softened, about 5 minutes. Add the garlic and cook for another minute.

Add the broccoli and stir to coat. Add the broth and simmer for 10 minutes, or until the broccoli has softened.

Working in batches, transfer the soup to an upright blender (or use an immersion blender) and mix until smooth. Transfer the soup back to the pot and add the remaining ½ teaspoon of salt.

Serve immediately, or allow to cool completely before transferring to an airtight container and storing in the fridge for up to 5 days. You can also freeze this soup for up to 6 months.

Makes about 1 quart

2 tablespoons olive oil or ghee

1 cup chopped yellow onion (from about half an onion)

1 teaspoon kosher sea salt, divided

1 large clove garlic, roughly chopped

3 heads of broccoli (about 1 pound total), stalks removed, cut into bite-size florets (about 3 cups total)

3 cups homemade Bone Broth (page 38) or store-bought broth (such as from Bonafide Provisions)

Swap It

For a vegan version, simply swap out the bone broth for vegetable broth or water.

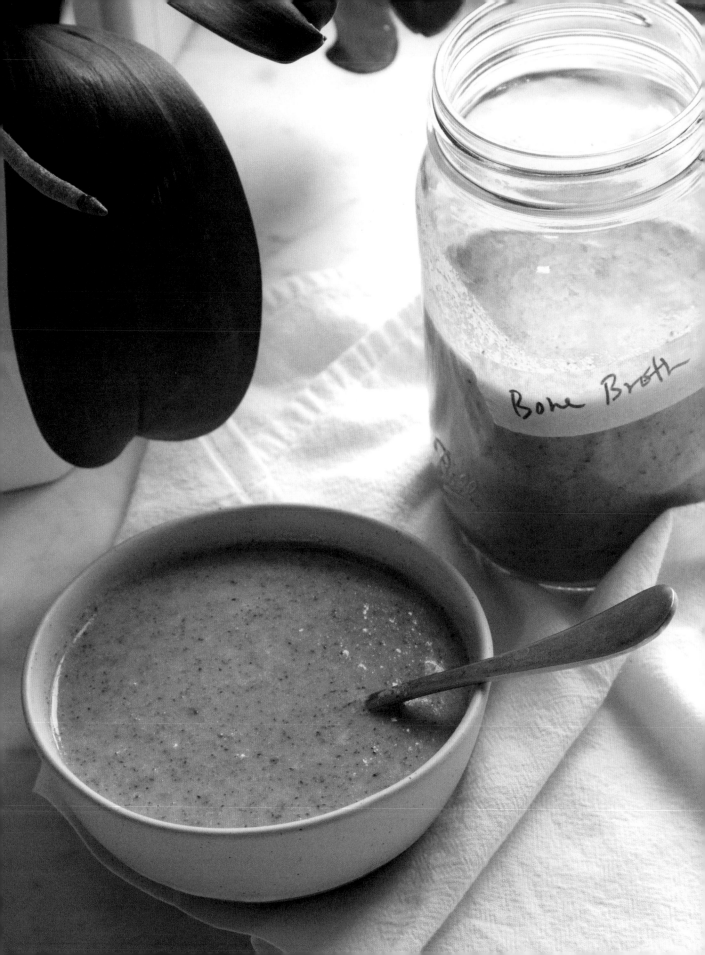

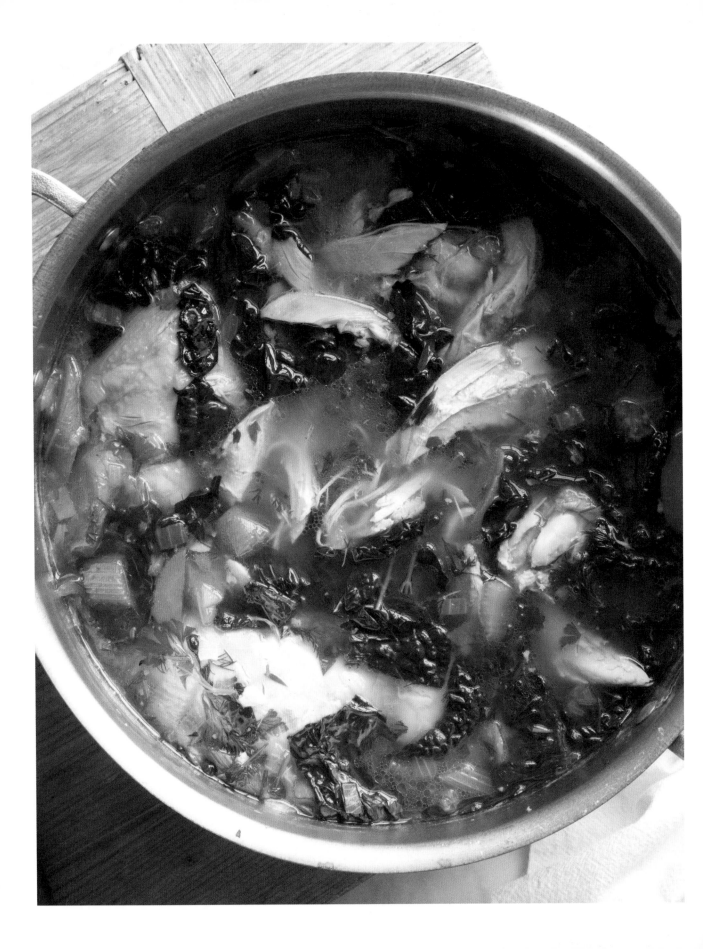

Rotisserie Chicken Soup

For me, this is a superior chicken soup recipe for two reasons: it comes together faster than the classic version because the chicken is already cooked, and the flavors are more concentrated from prior roasting. If you've never used a pre-roasted chicken in your soup before, you're going to be shocked at how delicious and developed these flavors are. You can use your own Overnight Roast Chicken (page 174) or pick up an herb-roasted chicken from the market on your way home. The more flavors the better!

Heat a large soup pot over medium for about 3 minutes. Add the ghee, reduce the heat to medium-low, and add the onions, carrots, celery, and ½ teaspoon of the salt. Stir to combine and sauté until softened, about 8 minutes, covering the pot to sweat the vegetables if they start to look dry. Add the garlic and stir for another minute.

Add the chicken, breaking it up into a few (bone-in) pieces as you go so that it fits into the pot, then add the bay leaves, water, and remaining 1½ teaspoon of salt. Stir and simmer, about 10 minutes. Partially cover and cook for 30 more minutes.

Stir in the kale and fresh herbs, then turn off the heat and serve immediately, bones and all.

Serves 6 to 8

3 tablespoons ghee

1 yellow onion, roughly chopped

4 carrots, roughly chopped

4 celery ribs, roughly chopped

2 teaspoons kosher sea salt, divided

4 large cloves garlic, minced

1 organic rotisserie chicken (about 3 pounds)

2 bay leaves (fresh or dried)

2½ quarts water

3 ounces chopped fresh kale or spinach (from 1 small bunch)

Handful of chopped fresh dill

Handful of chopped fresh flat-leaf parsley

Tip
You can add a roughly diced large zucchini a few minutes before you turn off the heat to bulk up the vegetables, and/or serve over a bowl of cooked rice or noodles to add starch.

Awase Dashi

Dashi is a family of stocks in Japanese cuisine that uses either one ingredient or a combination of a few to make a simple and flavorful broth centered around umami. The most common ingredients are kombu (kelp seaweed), *katsuobushi* (dried bonito), shiitake mushrooms, and *niboshi* (small dried fish). *Awase* means "to combine," so this recipe is a combination of two of the most common ingredients, kombu and katsuobushi.

This is a very simple preparation full of deep, savory flavor. It's a lovely healing broth that can be sipped on its own or used as a base for various miso, seafood, and noodle soup recipes. The seaweed adds minerals and iodine to the broth, making it great for thyroid support and nourishment.

This broth should never reach a full boil while the kelp or bonito flakes are still in it because these ingredients can turn bitter and viscous if they get too hot. Once you have strained the soup, you can of course boil it if necessary.

Using a damp cloth, wipe the kelp clean, then place it in a bowl with the cold water and leave in the fridge overnight to soak. Alternatively, you can soak the kelp for just 30 minutes in advance if you are short on time. Soaking longer will add more flavor.

Transfer both the kelp and water to a saucepan. Cook over medium heat until simmering, about 7 minutes, then discard the kelp. Heat the pot again, and when it's just barely simmering, add the bonito flakes, then turn off the heat. When the bonito flakes sink to the bottom of the pot, after about 10 minutes, strain the broth through a fine-mesh sieve into a bowl. Discard the bonito flakes. Enjoy immediately, or allow to cool and transfer to an airtight container and store in the fridge for up to 3 days.

Serves 2 to 4

1 (4-inch) square piece of kombu (about ½ ounce)

1 quart cold water

1 ounce dried bonito flakes (about 2 cups)

Tip
Once you've strained the broth, you can make a quick soup by adding 1 cup of sliced mushrooms or tender greens, or simply top with a handful of sliced green onions. You can also add some of your favorite cooked noodles or a serving of leftover cooked seafood, like salmon or shrimp, for a more complete meal.

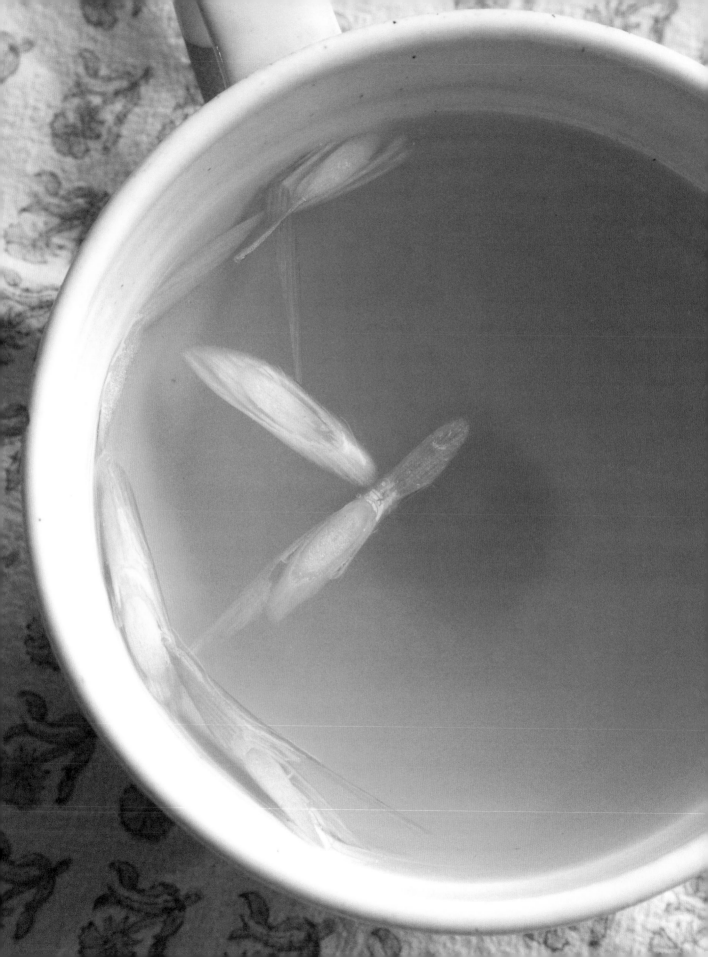

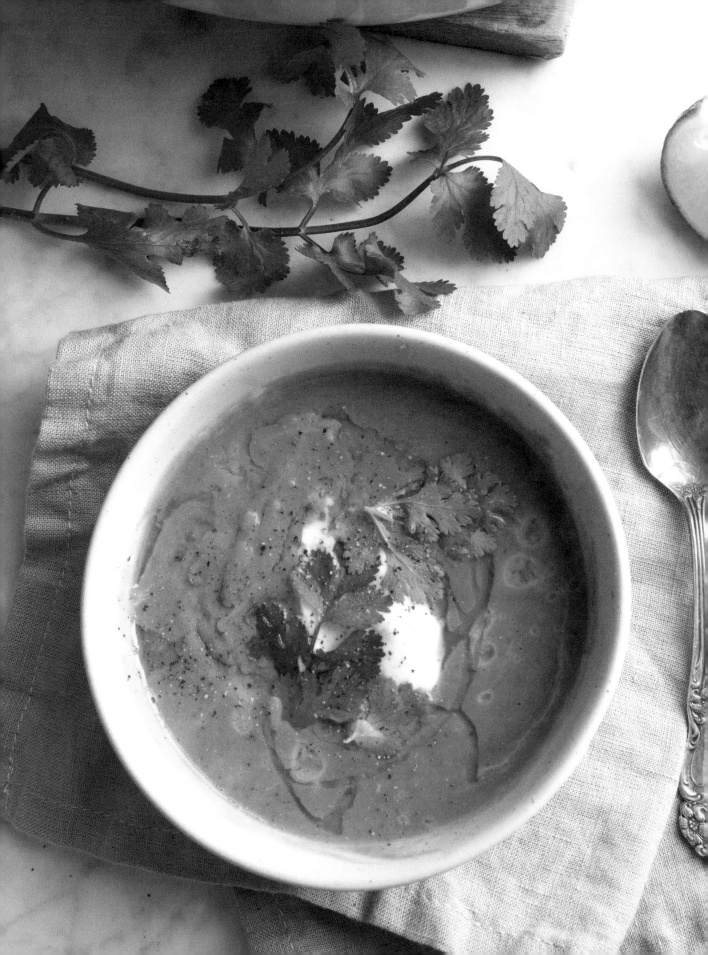

Red Lentil Mulligatawny Soup

When I was a kid, my dad and I would eat at an Indian restaurant called Mitali East on East Sixth Street in New York City, which was known as Curry Row. We ate there for 20 years. My husband even took my dad there to ask for his blessing to marry me. I always ordered the same things: poori, chicken korma (page 100), and mulligatawny soup. Many versions of this soup have emerged over the centuries, but most include a broth of some kind (chicken, beef, lamb, or vegetable) enriched with cream or coconut milk and also rice, lentils, or vegetables. My version uses chicken Bone Broth (page 38) for extra nourishment, lentils, and Fresh Almond Cream (page 16). This fragrant soup is sweet, creamy, rich, and absolutely easy to make.

For a heartier version, you can add 2 cups of cooked, shredded chicken thigh meat when you add the lentils.

Heat a medium Dutch oven over medium-low for about 3 minutes. Add the ghee, onions, carrots, celery, and 1 teaspoon of the salt and sauté for about 20 minutes, stirring occasionally, until the vegetables are very soft and only slightly browned. You can partially cover with a lid during cooking to slow the browning process, if needed.

Add the garlic, ginger, and spices and cook for 1 minute to toast and bloom the flavors. Add the lentils and cook for another minute. Add the broth and remaining ½ teaspoon of salt and bring to a gentle simmer, stirring occasionally, then cook, partially covered, until the lentils have softened, about 12 minutes.

Using a ladle, scoop half the soup into an upright blender and mix on low for 10 seconds. Return this mixture back to the pot and stir to combine. Add the almond cream and stir again. (To work ahead, you can cool and refrigerate the soup up to 3 days in advance, and reheat it over low, adding a splash of water as needed to loosen the soup.)

Serve in soup bowls with a dollop of yogurt, a drizzle of olive oil, a few cilantro leaves, and a wedge of fresh lime.

Serves 4

- ¼ cup ghee
- ½ yellow onion, chopped
- 2 medium carrots, chopped
- 2 large stalks of celery, chopped
- 1½ teaspoons kosher sea salt, divided
- 3 large cloves garlic, finely minced
- 1-inch piece of ginger, peeled and grated
- 1 tablespoon curry powder
- 1 teaspoon ground coriander
- 1 cup dry red lentils
- 6 cups chicken bone broth (see Bone Broth, page 38) or vegetable broth
- ½ cup Fresh Almond Cream (page 16)
- Dollop of unsweetened, plain Greek-style coconut yogurt (such as Cocojune Pure Coconut)
- Extra-virgin olive oil, for serving
- Small handful of torn, fresh cilantro leaves, for serving
- 1 lime, quartered, for serving

Swap It

You can substitute diced sweet potato for the carrot for extra sweetness. Regular chicken broth, beef, or vegetable broth would work well in place of the chicken bone broth.

Clams with Ginger-Coconut Broth

A big steaming pot of brothy clams and vegetables in a rich fragrant sauce of ghee, coconut milk, fish sauce, and lemongrass is one of my true pleasures. This dish is definitely Thai-influenced, but I've layered it with extra sweetness and depth from fennel, shallots, clam juice, and white wine. Once the clams have been cooked, I like to pile them onto a bed of white rice and ladle spoonfuls of the veggie-packed broth on top.

Start by cleaning the clams: Fill up a very large bowl with a gallon of cold water, add the sea salt, and stir to dissolve. Add the clams and place the bowl in the fridge for 30 minutes to an hour. Remove the clams from the fridge and set the bowl next to the sink. Don't drain the clams. Place a strainer in the sink. Two at a time, pluck the clams from the bowl, scrub them under cold running water using a stiff bristle brush, and drop them into the strainer.

Heat a large pot with a lid or Dutch oven over medium-low. Add the ghee; when melted, add the celery, fennel, shallots, garlic, and a pinch of salt. Cook gently until the vegetables soften and become fragrant, 5 to 7 minutes, stirring occasionally.

Add the wine and simmer for 5 minutes. Add the clam juice, coconut milk, fish sauce, ginger, lemongrass, coconut sugar, and lime leaves. Bring to a boil, then simmer for 15 minutes.

Add the clams, cover the pot with the lid, and cook until all the clams have opened, 8 to 10 minutes. Discard any clams that haven't opened. Fish out and discard the lemongrass and any leaves. Sprinkle with cilantro and green onions, then serve immediately in bowls filled with rice.

Serves 2 to 4

- ⅓ cup kosher sea salt, plus more for seasoning
- 3½ pounds littleneck or Manila clams (about 50 clams), scrubbed
- 5 tablespoons ghee
- 1 cup thinly sliced celery (from 2 to 3 stalks)
- 1 cup thinly sliced fennel (from 1 large bulb)
- 1 cup thinly sliced shallots (from 3 large shallots)
- 5 cloves garlic, thinly sliced
- 1 cup dry white wine
- 1 cup clam juice
- 1 cup full-fat coconut milk
- 1 tablespoon fish sauce
- ¾-inch piece of fresh ginger, sliced into ⅛-inch coins
- 1 lemongrass stalk (white and light-green part only), smashed a few times with the back of a knife
- 1 tablespoon coconut sugar
- 2 fresh lime leaves or bay leaves
- ½ cup roughly chopped cilantro
- ½ cup thinly sliced green onions
- White rice, for serving

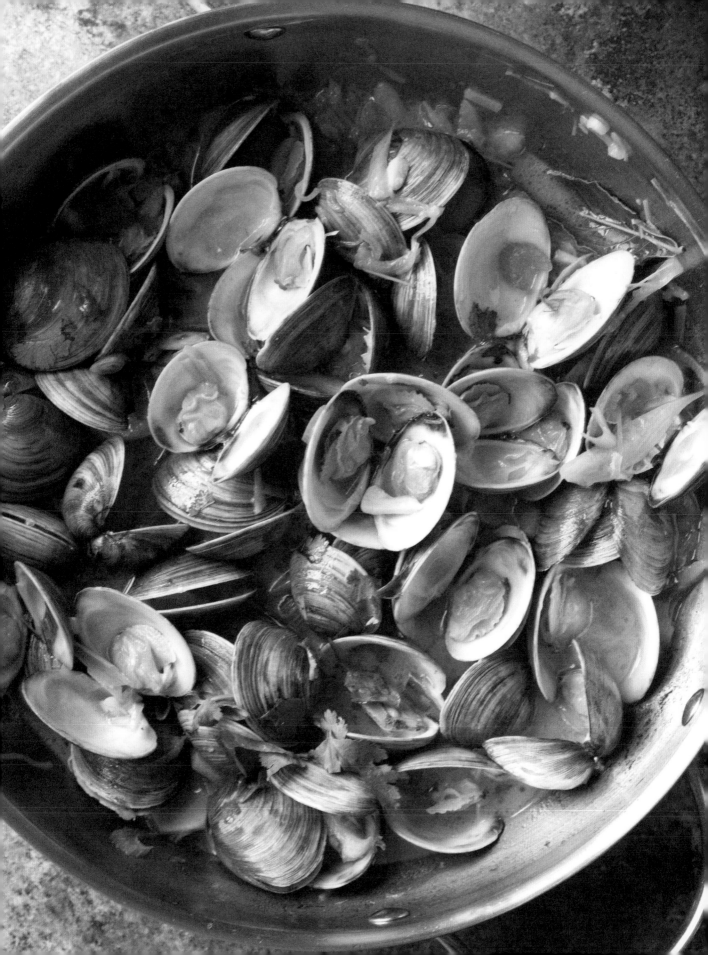

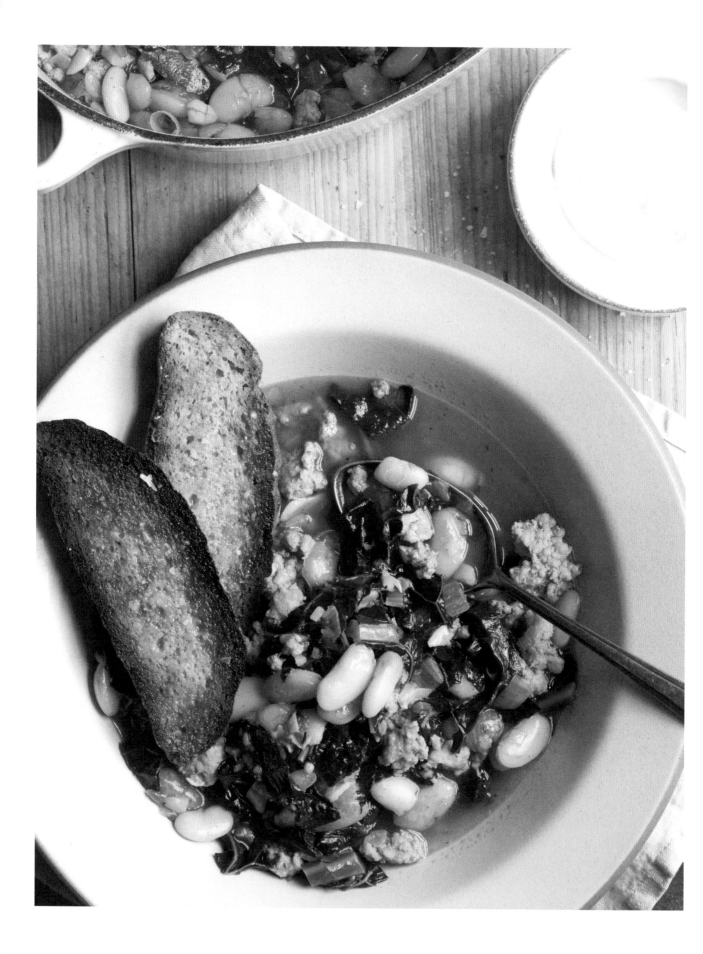

White Bean + Chorizo Stew

Instead of using store-bought chorizo sausage, I prefer to buy the components separately and use them to build the soup so the chorizo flavor permeates the broth. This way, I have much more control as to what goes into the pot and my body. Premade sausages can be filled with preservatives, "natural flavors," and spices that cause stomach upset for some of us. This spice blend can be customized for your needs, and don't worry: if you do leave something out of the recipe, it will still be delicious! Soups and stews are forgiving—that's part of their appeal. This is one giant, cozy pot! Serve with a toasted slice of the Grain-Free Vegan Boule (page 201) rubbed with some garlic and olive oil. It is the ultimate comfort dish on a cold winter night.

Heat a large Dutch oven over medium. Add 2 tablespoons of the olive oil, the ground meat, and 1 teaspoon of the salt. Brown the meat, breaking it apart with a large spoon and stirring occasionally, about 5 minutes. Using a slotted spoon, transfer the meat to a dish.

In the same pot, over medium heat, add the remaining 2 tablespoons of olive oil, the onions, the remaining ¾ teaspoon of salt, and black pepper. Sauté until soft and translucent, 7 to 8 minutes. Add the garlic and spices and cook for another minute, stirring constantly.

Add the beans, broth, fresh thyme, and bay leaves and stir to combine. Simmer for 10 minutes.

Add the kale and cook until it has wilted down, about 2 minutes. Add the meat back to the stew and simmer for another few minutes. Taste and adjust seasoning if necessary.

To dish up, ladle the stew into wide soup bowls, tuck some garlic toast on the side, drizzle with olive oil, and serve immediately.

Serves 4 to 6

- 4 tablespoons extra-virgin olive oil, divided, plus extra for toast and serving
- 1 pound ground organic pork, turkey, or lamb
- 1¾ teaspoons kosher sea salt, divided, plus extra for seasoning
- 1 large yellow onion, diced
- Freshly ground black pepper
- 5 large cloves garlic, minced
- 1 teaspoon ground paprika
- 1 teaspoon ground cumin
- ½ teaspoon dried oregano
- ½ teaspoon dried thyme
- ½ teaspoon dried coriander
- ½ teaspoon ground cardamom
- ½ teaspoon cinnamon
- 3 cups cooked cannellini beans (from Big Batch of Beans, page 40) or 2 (15.5-ounce) cans cannellini beans, rinsed and drained
- 3 cups chicken Bone Broth (page 38) or store-bought broth (such as from Bonafide Provisions)
- 3 sprigs of fresh thyme
- 2 bay leaves (fresh or dried)
- 1 (9-ounce) bunch of Tuscan kale, roughly chopped
- Grain-Free Vegan Boule garlic toast slices (see Tip on page 201), for serving

Black Friday Korma

I bring to you a childhood favorite: a mild, creamy, and velvety curry that we always eat on Black Friday. The day after Thanksgiving usually leaves us with a fridge full of leftovers. While making turkey sandwiches slathered in cranberry sauce is customary, I prefer to throw all the meat into a big pot and make a rich, fragrant shortcut korma, which is a mild curry braise of meat cooked in a thick sauce of yogurt, onions, nuts, and spices. Since it starts with cooked meat, we just make this gorgeous sauce, then mix everything and simmer. It's so easy. Any meat will do; you can use leftover turkey, chicken, or lamb. And if you're in the mood to make this another day of the year, a rotisserie chicken works beautifully, too. The key here is to slow-cook the onions until they are deep brown and caramelized. Don't rush this step! It adds crucial sweetness and depth to the sauce.

Heat a medium heavy-bottomed pot over medium. Add 3 tablespoons of the ghee, the onions, and the salt and sauté until the onions are golden brown, about 20 minutes. Stir in ¼ cup of the almonds and then turn off the heat. Let cool for 10 minutes; then transfer the mixture to an upright blender, add the yogurt, and blend until almost smooth, about 30 seconds.

Return the pot back to the stove and heat over medium-low. Add the remaining 2 tablespoons of ghee and the garlic and ginger. Sauté for 1 minute, until softened but not yet browning, then add the curry powder and cinnamon. Cook for another minute to bloom the spices. Stir in the turkey and sauté for a few more minutes, until the meat is evenly coated with the spices.

Add the yogurt mixture to the pot along with the water and mix everything together. Cover and simmer for 15 minutes. Season to taste.

Heat a small dry skillet over medium-high and toast the remaining ¼ cup of almonds until golden brown, 2 to 3 minutes.

Serve the curry immediately over bowlfuls of fluffy white rice, garnished with a sprinkle of toasted almonds and some freshly chopped cilantro.

Serves 4

5 tablespoons ghee, divided

2 cups chopped yellow onions (from 1 large onion)

½ teaspoon kosher sea salt, plus more for seasoning

½ cup blanched slivered almonds, divided

1 cup unsweetened, plain Greek-style coconut yogurt (such as Cocojune Pure Coconut)

4 large cloves garlic, finely minced

1½-inch piece of fresh ginger, finely minced

1 tablespoon ground curry powder

½ teaspoon ground cinnamon

1½ pounds cooked turkey, chicken, or lamb, pulled into bite-size pieces

1 cup water

¼ cup roughly chopped cilantro leaves, for garnish

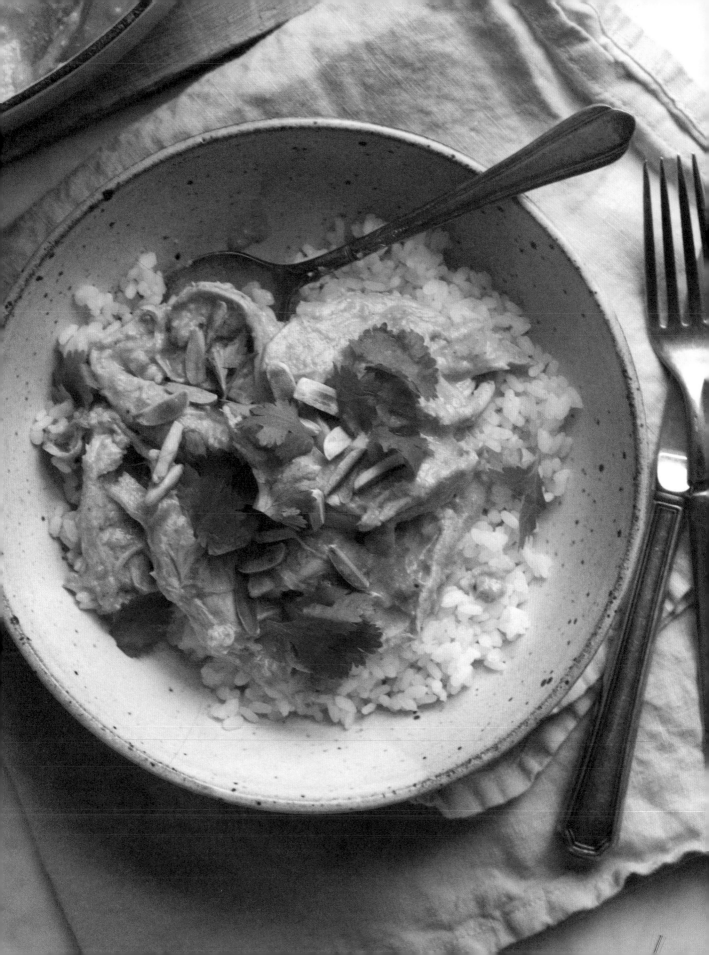

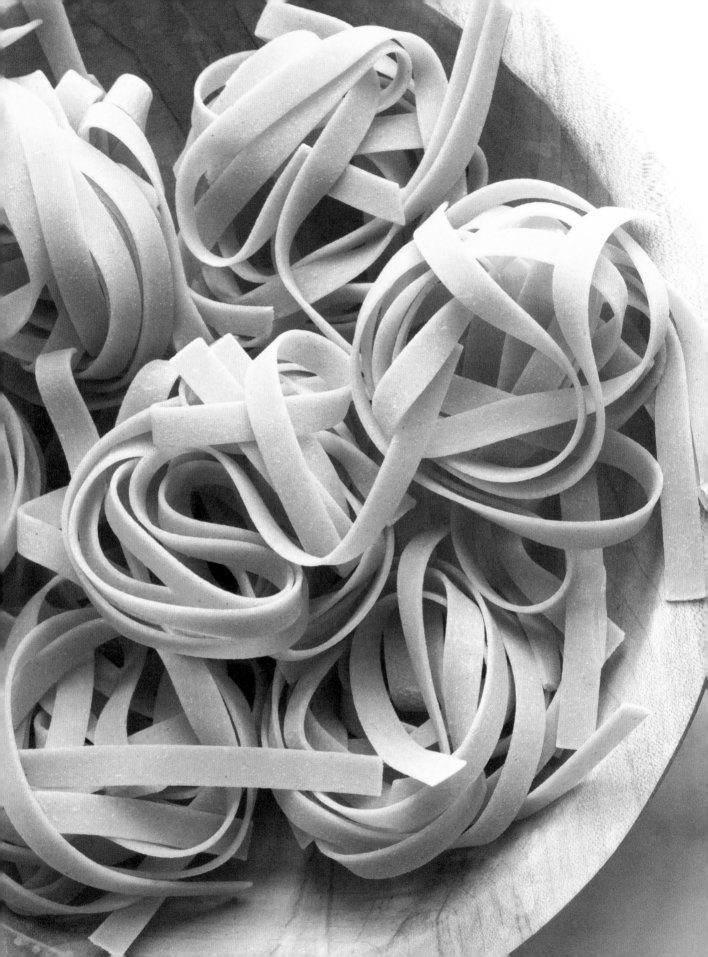

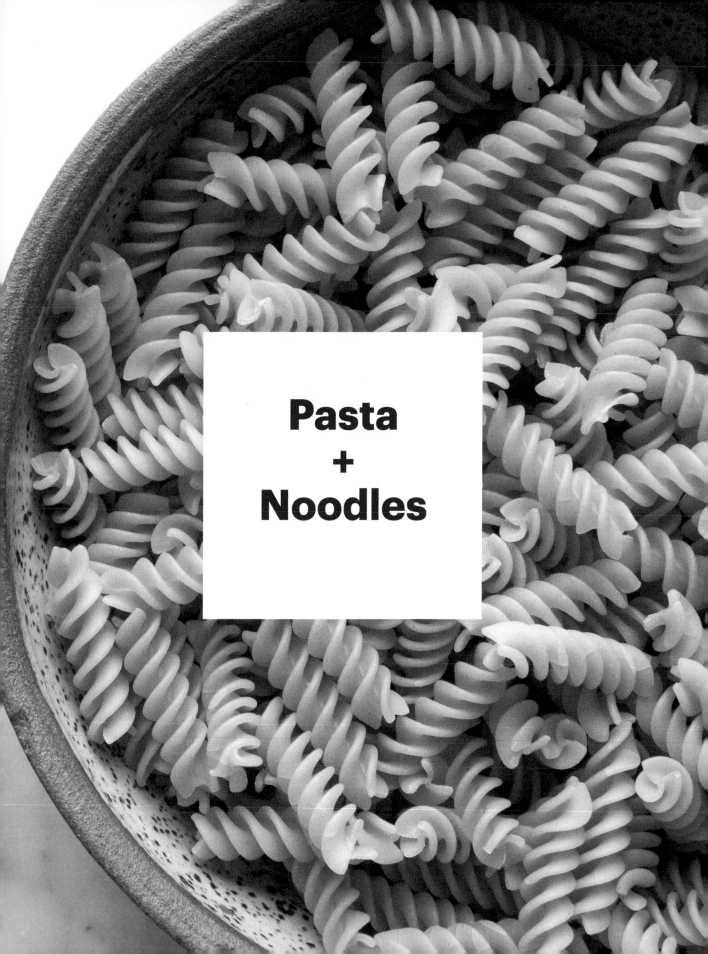

Pasta
+
Noodles

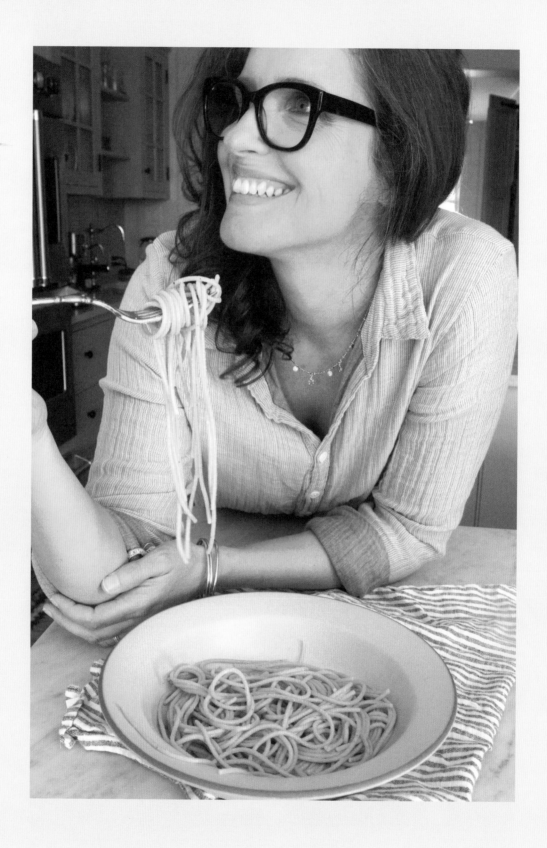

Stop Apologizing

In the early days of my health journey, I often found myself in situations where I ate things that I knew might cause me discomfort because I didn't have the right words to politely decline or I simply wasn't prepared and just very hungry! Today, I make sure to have something small before I head out into the unknown, so I'm not stuck eating foods that might cause problems. None of us want to ask our hosts to jump through hoops to make us the "right" dinner, but we can't sacrifice our health either. There will always be those people who roll their eyes when they discover you have dietary considerations that go outside the norm. There will also be people (and restaurants) who are very happy to accommodate your requests, too. In fact, sometimes a host is relieved to know how they can help and will appreciate your guidance. Stop apologizing for taking care of yourself, and instead, learn to be creative.

When we have guests over, I love the challenge of unifying a meal. I have to get stealthy and find ways to bridge the gaps between my own needs and the desires of my guests. I've got it down pretty well and usually make a few dishes that bring the table together. I keep it simple. For example, I make a big bowl of Tagliatelle Bolognese (page 110) and use a killer gluten-free pasta that none of my guests would suspect because it's a fantastic product. I cook it al dente and smother it in the sauce and serve it with a hunk of fresh Parmesan cheese on the side. To accompany this, I like to make Garlicky Greens with Apple Cider Vinegar (page 131) or a fresh salad with Marlit's Vinaigrette (page 8). I lay out snacks that are easily assembled from store-bought goods like fresh goat cheese, crunchy gluten-free crackers (the kind that even gluten-eaters love to eat, such as Mary's Gone Crackers brand), olives, crisp veggies, and Smashed Cumin Guacamole (page 22). Snacks are a great place to accommodate multiple eating styles because they are deconstructed and can be a combination of homemade and store-bought ingredients. When I'm hosting, my food doesn't stand out as "allergen-friendly" because I don't make any announcements and I choose familiar dishes that are delicious to everyone in my circle. As far as guests are concerned, I've made a pasta dinner with plenty of cheese available and a simple side dish, but it's something delicious that works for my body, too.

Penne alla Rosé

Unlike its sister, *penne alla vodka*, this spin-off uses rosé and fresh sweet cherry tomatoes instead of canned tomatoes. You can make this year-round, but it will be SO MUCH better if the tomatoes are in season, when your garden or local markets are overflowing with them. This version came together perfectly one summer night when there was an abundance of sweet cherry tomatoes in our garden, some leftover rosé, and a bowl of Fresh Almond Cream (page 16) in the fridge. Truly delicious, kid- and adult-friendly, and a celebration of summer in a bowl.

Heat a medium Dutch oven or large saucepan with a lid over medium-low. Add the ghee, onions, and a pinch of salt and sauté, uncovered, until the onions are soft and translucent, about 10 minutes. Stir occasionally, lowering the heat if necessary to prevent the onions from browning. Add the garlic and cook for a few more minutes, until it has softened.

Add the cherry tomatoes, salt, and rosé, and stir everything together. Simmer for 15 to 20 minutes, stirring occasionally, until the sauce has reduced and thickened slightly. Stir in the cream and transfer the mixture to an upright blender and mix until smooth. Return the sauce to the pot and cover with a lid to keep warm.

Bring a large stockpot of generously salted water to a boil. Add the pasta to the boiling water and cook until a little short of al dente, about 2 minutes less than the package instructs. Scoop out about 1 cup of pasta water before draining. Drain the pasta and carefully transfer it directly to the pot of sauce. Gently reheat the pasta and sauce together, making sure to coat the pasta well and finish cooking it, stirring in the reserved pasta water in ¼ cup increments if the sauce becomes too thick. Taste and adjust seasoning if necessary.

Serve the pasta in bowls, finished with fresh black pepper, torn basil, and a teaspoon (or to taste) of nutritional yeast if using.

Serves 4

3 tablespoons ghee

1 medium onion, diced

3 large cloves garlic, thinly sliced

2 pounds cherry tomatoes (about 2 pints), halved

¾ teaspoon kosher sea salt, plus more for seasoning

½ cup rosé

½ cup Fresh Almond Cream (page 16)

1 pound gluten-free penne (or any other short pasta of your choice)

Freshly ground black pepper (optional)

Fresh basil, for garnish

Nutritional yeast (optional)

Swap It

For a completely vegan sauce, substitute extra-virgin olive oil for the ghee. Also, for those who might want it, you could serve a bowlful of grated Parmesan cheese on the side.

Tip

If you're not using peak-season cherry tomatoes, add 3 tablespoons of tomato paste to add sweetness. Just stir it into the cooked tomatoes and simmer an additional minute or two before adding the cream.

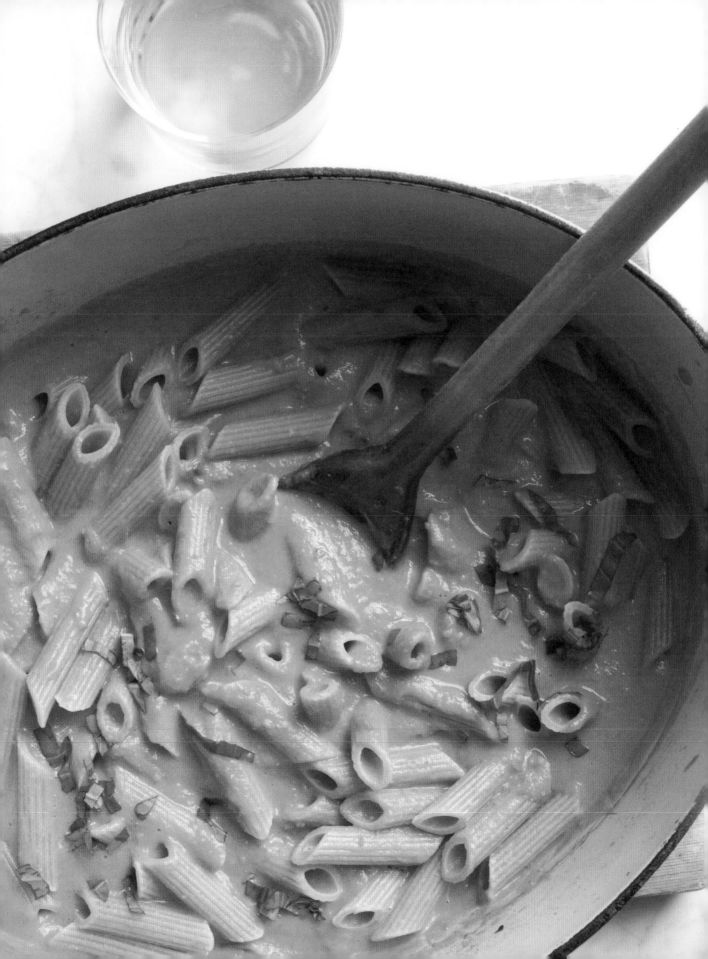

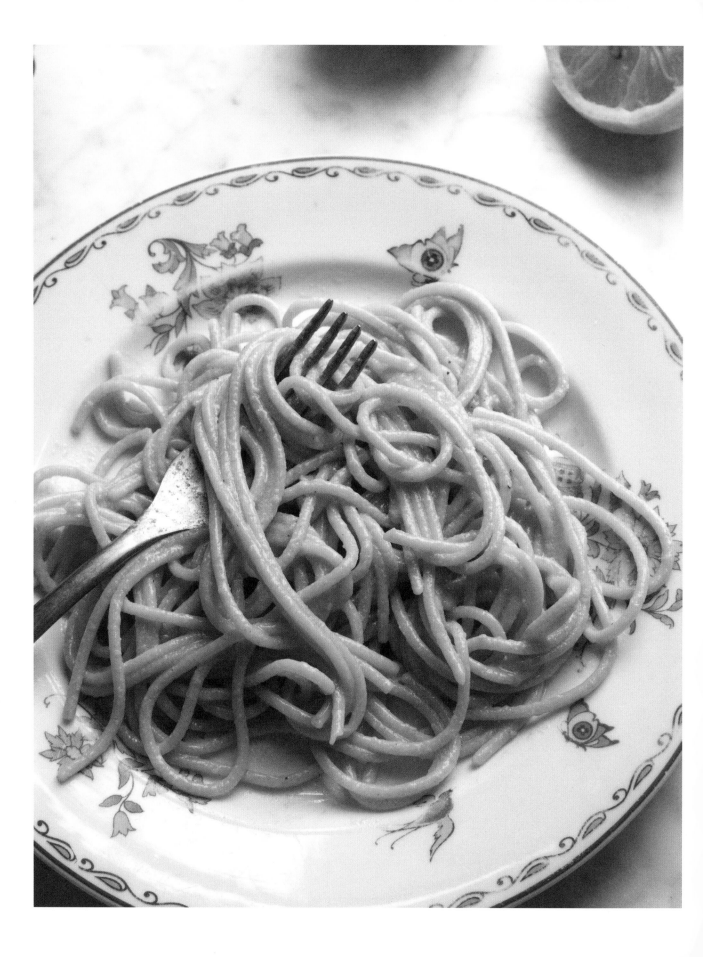

Lemon Spaghetti

I was first introduced to this dish in a NYC Italian restaurant on the Lower East Side. There is something so pure about the combination of spaghetti and lemon. The dish I knew was creamy, tangy, cheesy, and with perfectly al dente noodles . . . a deceptively simple meal, with really special flavor. Gone are the days of gluten and dairy for me, but I've managed to make a version that deeply satisfies my cravings for my old favorite, and my daughters have fully approved it. I usually have these ingredients on hand, so this is an easy dish to whip up when you have "nothing in the fridge." I use ghee instead of butter and nutritional yeast instead of cheese, paired with loads of fresh lemon zest and juice.

Bring a large stockpot of generously salted water to a boil. (It should taste like the ocean.) Add the pasta to the boiling water and cook until just short of al dente, about 2 minutes less than the package instructs. Reserve ½ cup of pasta water for the sauce, then drain the pasta.

Return the pasta to the pot and add the ghee. Zest the entire lemon directly into the pot, then cut it in half and squeeze the juice into the pot as well. Add the nutritional yeast and half the reserved pasta water. Using tongs, gently toss until the nutritional yeast has dissolved. Add the remaining pasta water and parsley and toss gently again until a creamy sauce has formed.

Serve immediately, straight from the pot. Finish with black pepper if using.

Serves 4

Kosher sea salt

1 (12-ounce) package gluten-free brown rice spaghetti (such as Jovial)

¼ cup ghee

1 large lemon

¼ cup nutritional yeast

⅓ cup roughly chopped flat-leaf parsley

Freshly ground black pepper (optional)

Tip
You can also serve with Parmesan cheese on the side.

Tagliatelle Bolognese

Ever since I was little, I've *loved* this dish. I don't eat pasta much anymore, but my kids and my husband do, and every now and then I will tuck into a bowl myself. Traditional Bolognese uses a combination of pork and beef, white wine, nutmeg, and milk. My version is simplified with a surprise spice. I use grass-fed ground beef, red wine, crushed fire-roasted tomatoes, a touch of tomato paste for added natural sweetness, and that surprise—a dash of cinnamon for warmth. It is such a cozy take on a classic comfort food. I kept the dose of cinnamon on the conservative side here, but feel free to add 1 whole teaspoon if you desire.

Heat a large, deep skillet with a lid over medium. Add the olive oil and onions and season with salt and pepper. Reduce the heat to medium-low and sauté until the onions are soft and translucent, 6 to 7 minutes. Add the garlic and cook for another minute, stirring. Add the ground beef, breaking it up with a spoon, increase the heat to medium, season with salt and pepper, and cook until the meat has browned, stirring and breaking it up as you go, about 4 minutes.

Add the wine and cook until most of the liquid has evaporated, stirring occasionally, 3 to 4 minutes. Add the crushed tomatoes, basil, oregano, cinnamon, and ½ teaspoon of the salt and stir to combine. Cover and simmer on low for 30 minutes, stirring occasionally, adding water if it starts to stick to the pan, ¼ cup at a time. When it has finished cooking, taste and adjust seasoning if necessary.

Bring a large stockpot of generously salted water to a boil. Add the pasta and cook according to the package instructions, until al dente. Scoop out about 1 cup of pasta water before draining.

Drain the pasta and add it directly to the skillet, tossing it with the sauce. If it is too thick, add a small splash of the reserved pasta water and gently stir to loosen it up. Divide the pasta evenly among shallow pasta bowls.

Alternatively, you can divide the drained pasta evenly between shallow pasta bowls and top it off with a few spoonfuls of sauce.

Serve immediately with the Parmesan cheese if using, or the topping of your choice.

Serves 4

- 2 tablespoons extra-virgin olive oil
- 1 medium red onion, diced
- ½ teaspoon kosher sea salt, plus more for seasoning
- Freshly ground black pepper
- 4 large cloves garlic, minced
- 1 pound grass-fed ground beef
- ½ cup dry red wine
- 1 (28-ounce) can fire-roasted crushed tomatoes
- ½ cup basil leaves, roughly chopped
- 1 teaspoon dried oregano
- ½ teaspoon ground cinnamon
- 1 (9-ounce) box gluten-free tagliatelle pasta (such as Jovial)
- Parmesan cheese, for serving (optional)

Swap It
Substitute a 9- to 12-ounce box of gluten-free pasta of your choice here, such as penne, spaghetti, fusilli, or farfalle. You can also substitute a bowl of Steak Knife Roasted Vegetables (page 122) for the pasta for a grain-free version.

Tip
Another way to eat Bolognese is as a warm appetizer. Set out a bowl of this sauce with crusty slices of toasted garlic bread (see Tip on page 201) for dipping and skip the pasta altogether!

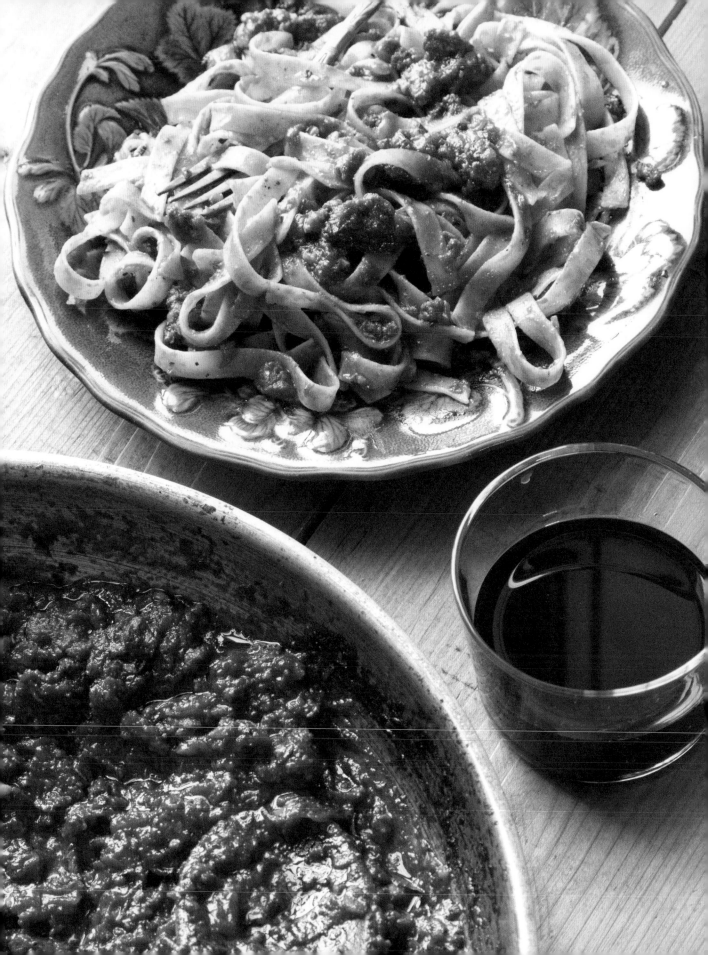

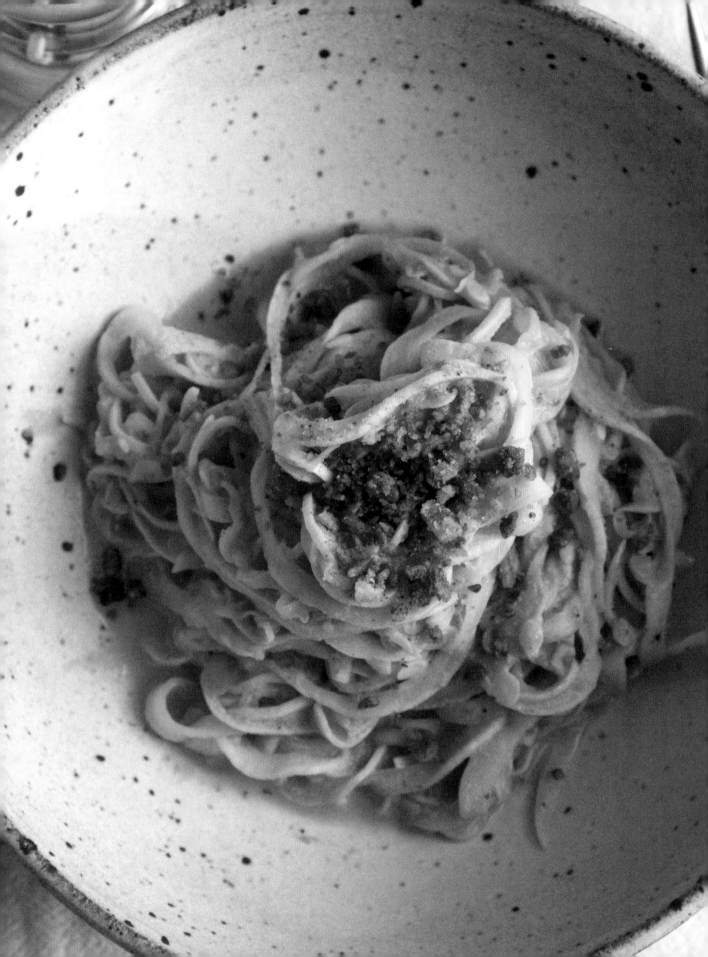

Cacio e Pepe 2.0

Dare I say that this version of *cacio e pepe* might stand up proud to the classic Roman dish? I'm sure the pasta police will have something to say about that, but I don't care. I've learned over the years how to substitute ingredients so I can enjoy classic recipes like this without suffering any consequences. Here I've swapped out pasta for tender yellow squash and replaced the cheese with nutritional yeast. Even if you're not on any kind of particular diet, this vegetable dish has tons of rich cheesy flavor, a super creamy texture, and the perfect crunch thanks to my Toasted Plantain Crumbs (page 37). It's also high in protein and B vitamins found naturally in nutritional yeast.

Tossing the squash in salt and allowing it to release its excess juices prior to cooking ensures that you won't end up with soggy noodles and a watered-down sauce. This recipe comes together very quickly, making it ideal for a last-minute side dish. Double it for a main course.

You will need a vegetable spiralizer to make the noodles or you can find them premade in the frozen vegetable section at the grocery store.

Start by tossing the "noodles" with the salt in a sieve set over a bowl. Allow the noodles to sit for 20 minutes; they will release their juices and drain.

Heat a large nonstick skillet over medium. Add the ghee and garlic and sauté for 30 seconds, until fragrant. Using tongs, add the noodles and toss to combine. Add the nutritional yeast and toss again until all the powder has dissolved. Don't worry if it looks dry, the nutritional yeast will become creamy within a few minutes.

Add the fresh black pepper and toss to make sure everything is mixed well. This dish will come together fast and should be very creamy.

Carefully transfer the noodles to each serving bowl, twisting each bundle with the tongs as you plate it up. Sprinkle the toasted crumbs on top and serve immediately.

Serves 2

2 medium-size yellow squash (about 1½ pounds total), spiralized

1½ teaspoons kosher sea salt

2 tablespoons ghee

1 large clove garlic, minced

3 tablespoons nutritional yeast

Freshly cracked black pepper

2 tablespoons Toasted Plantain Crumbs (page 37)

Tip
You can make this in advance and reheat it in a medium skillet with 1 to 2 tablespoons of water on medium-low.

Eggplant Moussaka Bake with Fresh Almond Ricotta

Inspired by the Greek dish moussaka, this layered lasagna-like bake substitutes whole slices of eggplant for the traditional pasta sheets, making a vegetable-packed, extra-hearty version that I actually think is better. The Fresh Almond Ricotta Cheese (page 15) perfectly enriches this dish without relying on dairy. For extra color and phytonutrients, I've also added a layer of sautéed spinach greens. Like most lasagna-style dishes, this takes a little time to prepare and requires a few pans, but it's worth the extra effort. This dish is so decadent, rich with layers of nourishment, and very filling. I make this every year during the holiday season when we're hosting family, always to rave reviews.

Preheat the oven to 425°F, and line 2 large baking sheets with parchment paper.

In a large bowl, toss the eggplant slices with ¼ cup of the olive oil and ½ teaspoon of the salt and transfer them to the baking sheets, spaced evenly apart. Roast in the oven for 35 minutes, until lightly golden. Remove from the oven.

Reduce the oven temperature to 375°F. Heat a large skillet over medium for about 3 minutes. Add 2 tablespoons of the olive oil, then add the onions and season with a pinch of salt. Sauté until softened, 5 to 7 minutes. Add about 6 cloves' worth of the minced garlic and cook for 1 minute, stirring. Add the beef and lamb and 1½ teaspoons of the salt and cook, breaking up the meat and stirring, until fully browned, about 8 minutes. Add the spices and cook for another few minutes. Add the can of crushed tomatoes and the tomato paste and stir everything to mix well. Season to taste and simmer for 5 minutes.

Heat a second medium skillet over medium for about 3 minutes. Add 1 tablespoon of the olive oil and the remaining garlic and sauté for 30 seconds. Add the spinach and remaining ½ teaspoon of the salt. Sauté until all the liquid has evaporated, about 8 minutes. Turn the heat off.

Serves 6 to 8

- 3 medium-size eggplants (about 2½ pounds), ends trimmed and sliced lengthwise into ¼-inch-thick slices
- ¼ cup extra-virgin olive oil plus 4 tablespoons, divided
- 2½ teaspoons kosher sea salt, plus more for seasoning
- 1 medium red onion, diced
- 7 large cloves garlic, minced and divided
- 1 pound grass-fed ground beef
- 1 pound grass-fed ground lamb
- 1 teaspoon dried basil
- 1 teaspoon dried oregano
- 1 teaspoon ground cinnamon
- 1 (28-ounce) can fire-roasted crushed tomatoes
- 3 tablespoons tomato paste
- 1 (16-ounce) bag frozen organic spinach
- 3 cups Fresh Almond Ricotta Cheese (page 15)

To assemble the bake, drizzle the remaining tablespoon of olive oil in the bottom of a 9-by-13-inch baking dish. Cover the bottom of the dish with a layer of eggplant. Spread 1 cup of ricotta cheese over the eggplant, then spoon about a third of the meat sauce over. Lay the second layer of eggplant over the sauce, followed by another cup of ricotta cheese. Carefully spread all the spinach evenly over the ricotta cheese. Spoon another third of the sauce over the spinach. Finally, arrange the last layer of eggplant, the last third of the sauce, and any remaining ricotta cheese on top.

Cover with aluminum foil and bake for 30 minutes. Remove the foil and continue to bake for another 20 minutes, until bubbling. If you want to crisp up the top further, you can broil on high for 4 to 5 minutes, or until crispy.

Allow the bake to rest for 10 minutes, then serve immediately.

Tip
Serve with Garlicky Greens with Apple Cider Vinegar (page 131). You can also make and refrigerate this up to 2 days in advance. It might even taste better this way! Reheat in a 350°F oven for 30 minutes, covered with foil.

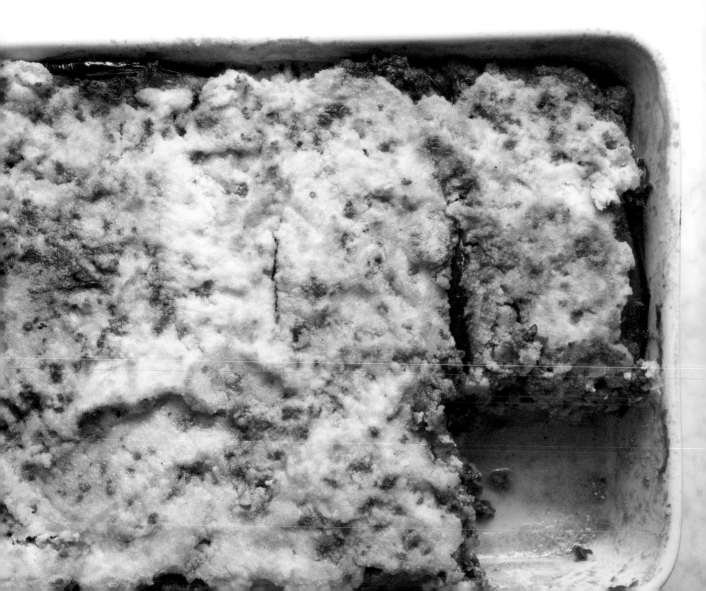

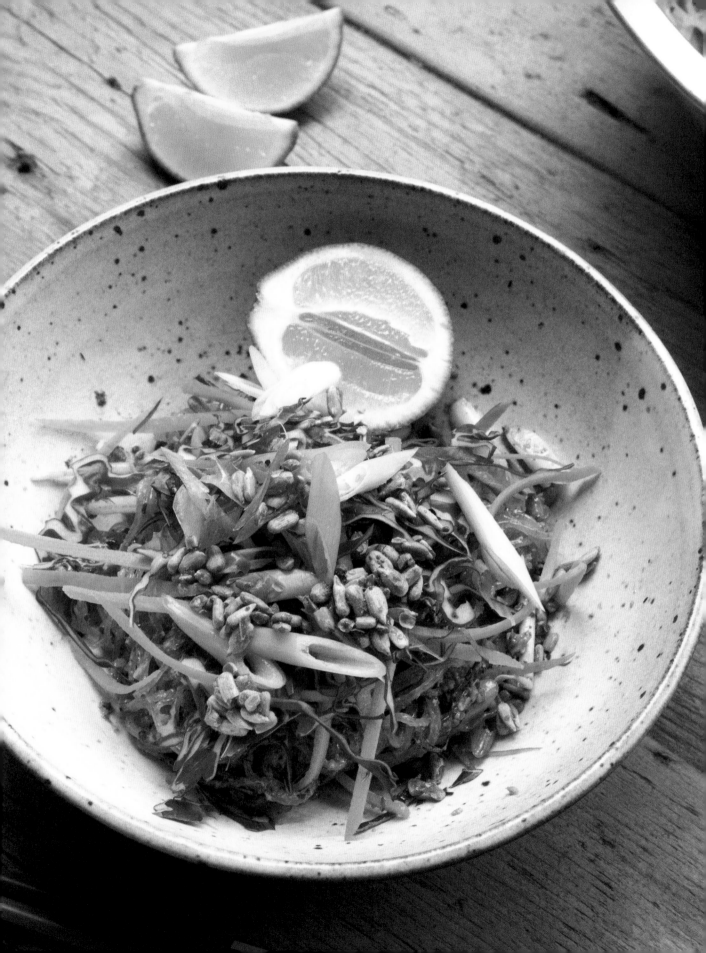

Creamy Pad Thai Kelp Noodles

Classic pad thai, made with rice noodles, is one of my favorite dishes to eat, but I know some people prefer to limit their grain intake, myself included. Kelp noodles are a great substitute because their slightly crunchy texture lends itself perfectly to the dish. Seaweed is also one of the best sources of dietary iodine, which helps support thyroid health. This dish is loaded with crispy veg, smothered in a vibrant and fresh creamy pesto, and topped off with sweet sunflower seeds. It's a cool and refreshing noodle dish that you could serve in the summer months alongside Whole Garlic Prawns with Charred Lemon (page 159).

Look for kelp noodles in the international or refrigerated sections of any large grocery store.

Rinse the kelp noodles under warm tap water in a colander in the sink, separating the noodles by hand. Once drained, transfer them to a medium mixing bowl and add the salt and enough hot water to cover the noodles. Swish around to dissolve the salt and allow to soak for 30 minutes. Transfer the noodles to a strainer to drain, and dry the mixing bowl.

Return the noodles to the mixing bowl and add the pesto. Toss the noodles, making sure to coat them well with the sauce. Add the carrots, cabbage, and sprouts and toss again to mix well.

Transfer the noodles to a serving bowl and top them off with the green onions and sunflower seeds. Serve immediately with lime wedges.

Serves 2

1 (12-ounce) bag kelp noodles (such as from Sea Tangle Noodle Company)

1 teaspoon kosher sea salt

1 cup Creamy Thai Pesto (page 11)

½ cup julienned or shredded carrots (from about 1 large carrot)

½ cup shredded purple cabbage

½ cup fresh bean sprouts

½ cup thinly sliced green onions

¼ cup Toasted Maple Sunflower Seeds (page 35)

Lime wedges, for serving

Swap It
You can substitute toasted almond slivers or peanuts for the sunflower seeds.

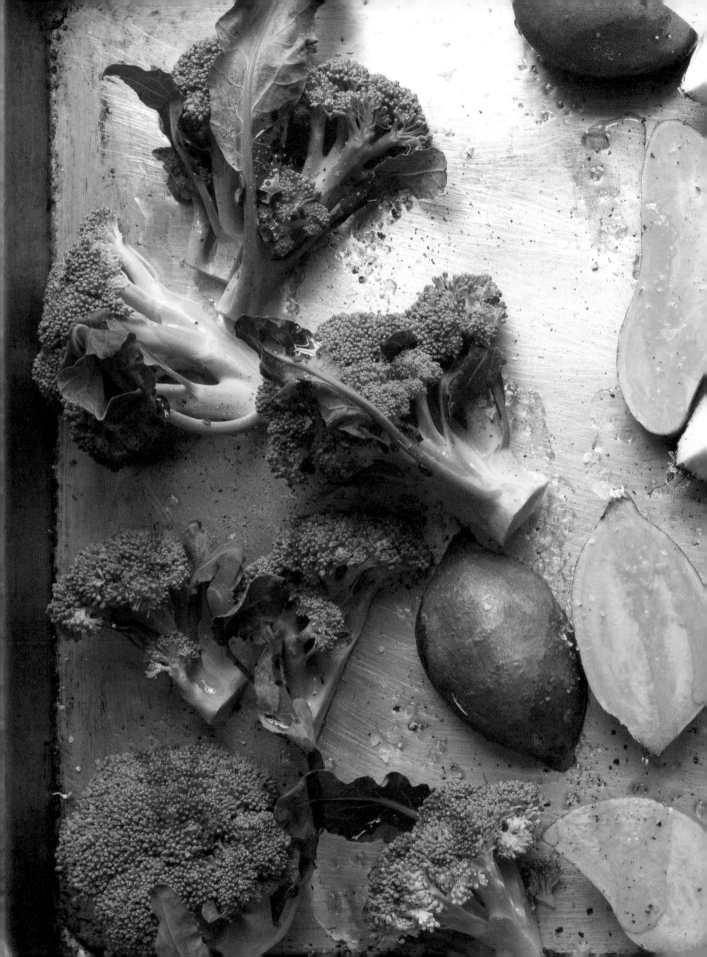

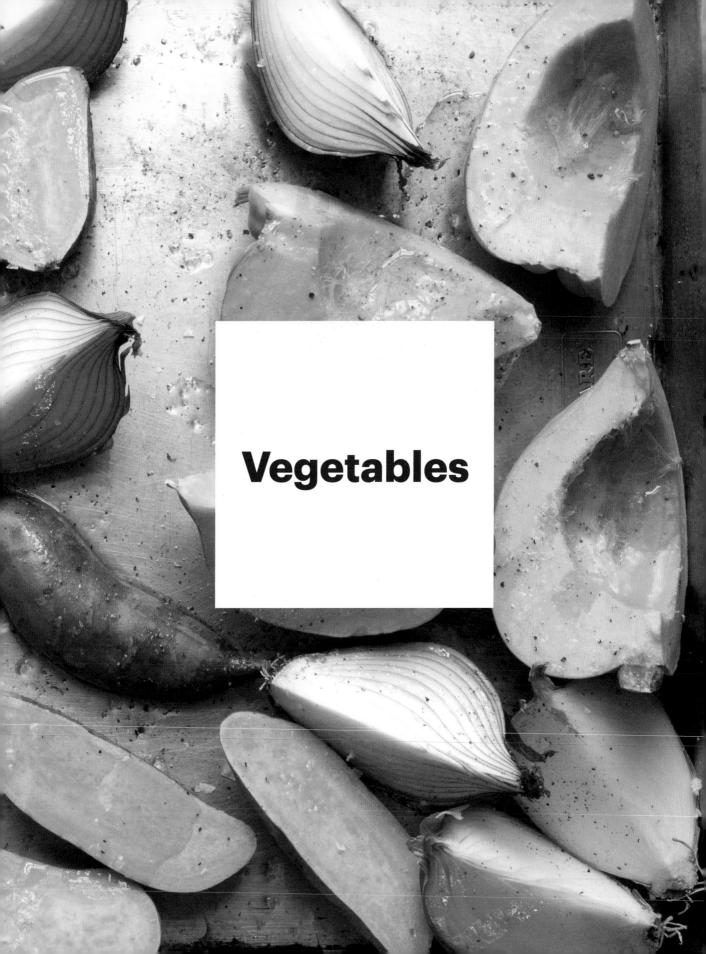

Vegetables

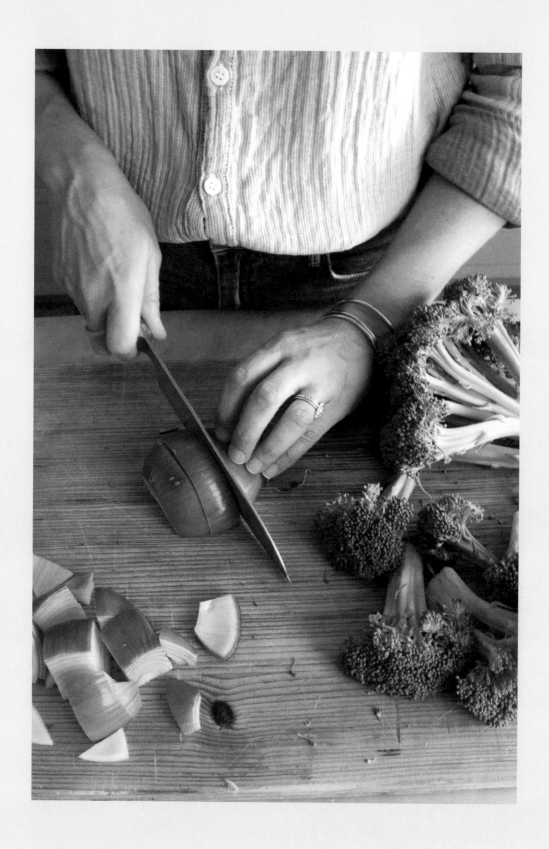

Cooking for Your Future Self

One of the hardest aspects of making changes to your health is figuring out what habits are actually sustainable. Often, we get so excited about the prospect of healing that we charge ahead with new diets and routines, only to discover that in our day-to-day lives these shifts don't always line up with our schedules, our budgets, or maybe the people around us. We want to, say, get enough protein and eat veggies with every meal, but we burn out. The key is finding small changes or habits that you can easily bring into your life that make a big impact. Instead of restricting yourself, look for foods that support your health in a positive way and crowd out the things that don't. Cooking for your future self—cooking one thing your body loves, but cooking more of it by doubling or tripling the recipe—is a great way to do this.

Every time you turn on the oven or stove to make something you enjoy that also loves you back, you have an opportunity to double up or make a big batch of food that can be used for future meals. This can be something as simple as rice (page 44) or a big pot of beans (page 40), or more of a project, like making two roast chickens (page 174), two loaves of bread instead of one (page 201), a larger batch of turkey patties (page 177), or extra roasted vegetables (page 122). Whenever you cook, ask yourself whether you can make more to somehow help your future self. This is a flexible practice that you can start today, and it doesn't ask you to change. It just means that tomorrow and the next day you'll have a little extra time to focus on your goals, knowing that your health is supported.

Steak Knife Roasted Vegetables

The most common question I get from people who are changing their diet is "What do I eat now if I'm removing gluten and grains?" Enter roasted vegetables. You can replace the grains in grain bowls with roasted vegetables, ladle Bolognese over them instead of pasta, toss them with pesto, throw them into salads, stuff them into wraps and omelets, drop them into soups, or turn them into purées. They are one of the easiest things to make and really support your health with tons of fiber, vitamins, and minerals. They help to detoxify your system and make you feel full and satiated. All you really need is olive oil and salt, but you can add 1 teaspoon of ground spices and herbs such as cumin, thyme, or sage or 1 tablespoon of fresh citrus zest to punch them up, too.

Following are some of my favorite vegetables, but you can really roast almost anything. A few things to know: You should cut all vegetables into pieces of roughly the same size so they roast evenly. You can leave the skin on squash and just eat it. Save the stalks of your broccoli and cauliflower for ricing (see Tip, next page). Truth be told, I don't wash my vegetables before I roast them because they never really crisp up as well. If you do wash them, make sure to dry them thoroughly, or they will steam instead of roast.

I line my baking sheets with parchment paper to ensure nothing sticks to the pan and give myself an easy cleanup. Alternatively, you can skip the parchment paper, throw the empty baking sheet into the oven for 15 minutes before roasting, toss your veggies in a large bowl with olive oil and salt, then dump them onto the preheated pan and pop it back into the oven. This will help get a head start on those crispy edges. You must play with this recipe until you get crispy and caramelized edges full of concentrated, irresistible flavor.

Finally, make sure to serve your vegetables with steak knives. This preparation calls for big hunks of veg that are hearty, and diners need the proper tools. Plus, it's more fun!

Non-Starchy Roasted Vegetables

Preheat the oven to 450°F, and line a large baking sheet with parchment paper.

In a large bowl, combine the vegetables, add the olive oil, salt, and pepper, and toss by hand until everything is well coated.

Pour the vegetables onto the prepared baking sheet and spread them out evenly in a single layer. Roast for 25 minutes, or until crisp and browned at the edges.

Serve immediately, or cool and store in an airtight container in the fridge for up to 3 days.

Serves 4 to 6

3 pounds non-starchy vegetables (such as a combination of broccoli, cauliflower, and red onion), cut into 3-inch florets and wedges, all roughly the same size

¼ cup extra-virgin olive oil

½ teaspoon kosher sea salt

Freshly ground black pepper

Tip
Take any leftover broccoli or cauliflower stalks and rice them by pulsing in a food processor until broken down. The resulting "rice" can be sautéed with a little olive oil, garlic, salt, and pepper and made into a flavorful rice substitute.

Starchy Roasted Vegetables

Preheat the oven to 425°F, and line a large baking sheet with parchment paper.

In a large bowl, combine the vegetables, add the olive oil, salt, and pepper, and toss by hand until everything is well coated.

Pour the vegetables onto the prepared baking sheet and spread them out evenly in a single layer. Roast for 30 minutes, or until crisp and browned at the edges.

Serve immediately, or cool and store in an airtight container in the fridge for up to 3 days.

Serves 4 to 6

3 pounds starchy unpeeled vegetables (such as delicata squash and sweet potatoes), cut into 3-inch pieces of roughly the same size and shape, seeds removed as necessary

¼ cup extra-virgin olive oil

½ teaspoon kosher sea salt

Freshly ground black pepper

Tips
Don't overcrowd the pan, because the vegetables need room to crisp up. If you need to, spread them out between two pans or roast them in batches.

Using tongs, place any cut side of the vegetables facing down to help them brown more evenly.

Crispy Brussels Sprouts with Fish Sauce Caramel

Yes, you read that correctly; you can make caramel using fish sauce! The sauce is traditionally used to bring color and sweetness to braises and stir-fries. My version uses maple syrup, fish sauce, and vinegar, which all reduce to a concentrated syrup that is sweet and salty and intensely delicious. If you're already on the fish sauce train, I'm happy for you. If not, don't be afraid! It's often misunderstood and thought of as fishy, but it's not. In this recipe it's more of a background flavor, used to build in savory, rich umami without the actual fishiness. This is everything you want in a Brussels sprouts dish; the caramelized burnt sprout edges make it so addictive. Also, I don't wash the sprouts beforehand because they will steam instead of crisp up.

Heat a small saucepan over medium. Add 1 tablespoon of the olive oil and the garlic. Reduce the heat to medium-low and cook for 1 minute, until fragrant, then add the maple syrup, fish sauce, and vinegar. Simmer for 8 to 10 minutes, until the sauce has reduced by about half and starts to get extra foamy. Transfer the sauce to a small bowl and allow to cool for 20 minutes, until the sauce thickens, stirring occasionally.

Place the Brussels sprouts in a medium mixing bowl, drizzle with 1 tablespoon of the olive oil, season with salt and lots of fresh pepper, and toss together well.

Heat a large skillet (preferably cast-iron) over medium-high until very hot. Add the remaining 3 tablespoons of olive oil, then add the Brussels sprouts, quickly turning them so their cut sides face down in the pan. Cook for about 3 minutes, or until charred and crisp, then flip over to cook for another 1 to 2 minutes, until browned.

Transfer the sprouts to a serving dish. Drizzle with ¼ cup of the sauce to start, and serve immediately. Serve the extra sauce on the side, or transfer to an airtight container and store in the fridge for another use.

Serves 2 to 4

5 tablespoons extra-virgin olive oil, divided

1 clove garlic, minced

½ cup maple syrup

¼ cup fish sauce

2 tablespoons apple cider vinegar

1 pound Brussels sprouts, trimmed and halved

Kosher sea salt

Freshly ground black pepper

Swap It
Substitute bite-size broccoli, cauliflower, zucchini, asparagus, or green beans for the Brussels sprouts.

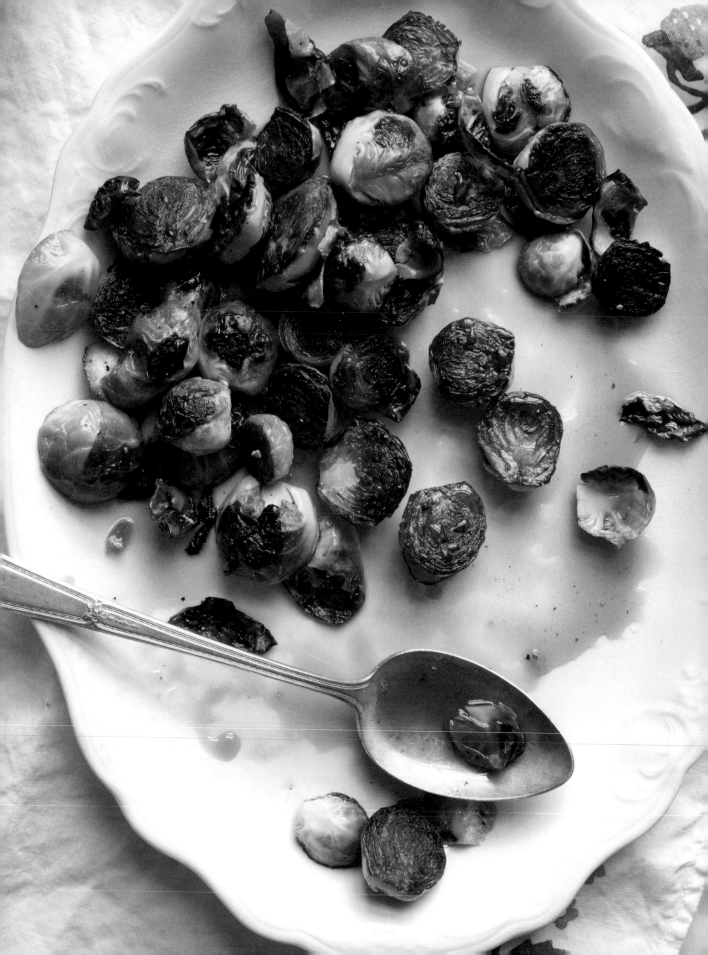

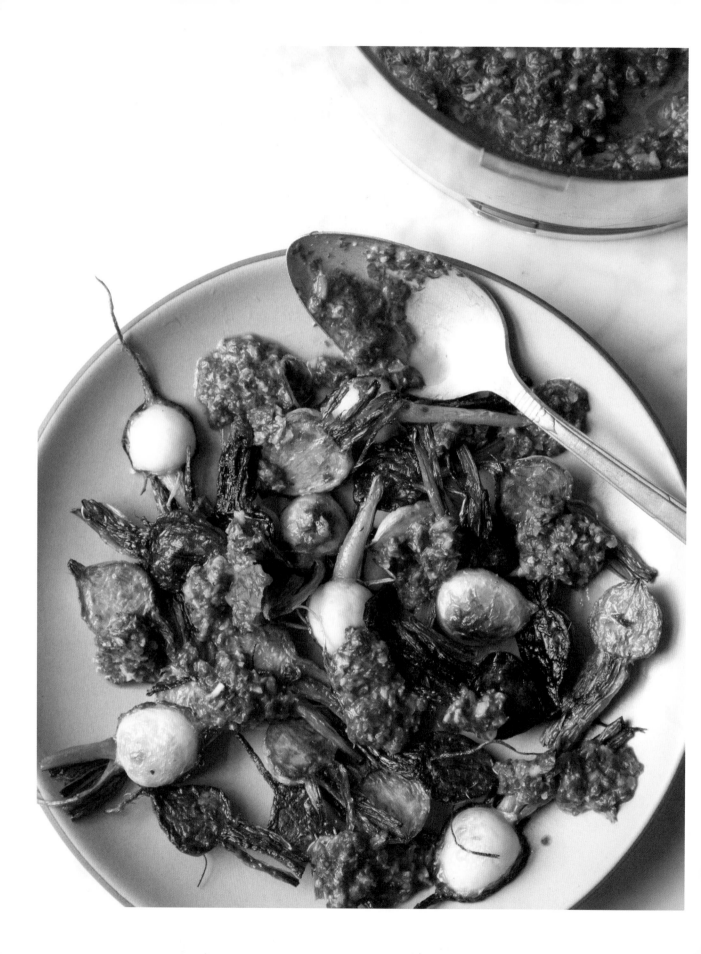

Pan-Sautéed Baby Turnips with Turnip Green Pesto

If you happen to see a fresh and lively bunch of beautiful baby turnips at the market, change your plans, grab them, and make this dish. They are sweet and tender with just a hint of nutty, earthy pepperiness. I love this recipe because we're using the entire vegetable, along with its leaves, tops, and tails. It's a zero-waste situation. And after preparing this dish, you will have plenty of a zesty, bright, flavorful pesto left over that you can serve on chicken, steak, or fish, or hold on to in the fridge to top future roasted veggies, use as a sandwich spread, or simply eat straight by the spoonful. I suggest making the pesto first because the turnips cook up quickly and it's nice to have the sauce ready to go!

You want to look for turnips that are small—close to radish size.

First, make the pesto: Combine the turnip greens, lemon zest and juice, garlic, pine nuts, anchovy fillets, and ¼ teaspoon of the salt in the bowl of a food processor and pulse a few times, until broken down and mixed well. Add the olive oil and pulse again, scraping down the sides if necessary, until it becomes a rustic sauce. Add more olive oil if needed, 1 tablespoon at a time, until loose enough to drizzle with a spoon. (You should have about 1 cup.)

Heat a cast-iron skillet over medium-high for about 5 minutes. We want this pan *hot*. Add the ghee; it should be smoking as it melts. Add the turnips and the remaining ¼ teaspoon of salt and give them a quick stir to coat everything evenly. Using tongs, turn each turnip cut side down. Cook for 1 minute, then reduce the heat to medium-low and continue cooking for 6 to 7 minutes, or until the turnips are crispy outside and tender inside. You should be able to pierce one easily with a small paring knife.

When they're done, transfer the turnips to a serving dish and drizzle with about half the pesto. Serve immediately.

Serves 2

1 bunch (about 1 pound) of baby turnips, greens trimmed and roughly chopped (about 2 packed cups greens), turnips halved lengthwise

Zest of 1 small lemon, plus 1 tablespoon juice

1 large clove garlic, roughly chopped

¼ cup toasted pine nuts (see Tip on page 25)

4 anchovy fillets, roughly chopped

½ teaspoon kosher sea salt, divided

⅓ cup extra-virgin olive oil, plus more as needed

2 heaping tablespoons ghee

Swap It
Substitute toasted pumpkin seeds or walnuts for the pine nuts. To make this vegan, substitute a teaspoon of miso paste for the anchovy in the sauce. In the pan, use olive oil instead of ghee.

Tip
To make this nut- or seed-free, simply omit the pine nuts from the recipe. You will still have a bright, zesty sauce.

Pan-Roasted Cauliflower with Caper-Currant Relish + Yogurt-Tahini Sauce

The first time I had some iteration of this Mediterranean-inspired dish was at a restaurant in New York City. We ordered a whole head of cauliflower that came deeply caramelized and roasted, served over a pool of tahini or yogurt (or maybe it was both?) and topped off with herbs, pistachios, and spices. We were left to cut it apart ourselves, dragging hunks of veg through all the different components on the plate. It was a religious experience. My version simplifies the cooking process a little by breaking down the vegetable into a few pieces that cook evenly together in a hot pan and includes my sweet-and-sour Caper-Currant Relish (page 25).

Preheat the oven to 400°F.

In a small bowl, whisk together all the ingredients for the Yogurt-Tahini Sauce.

In a large bowl, drizzle the cauliflower with ¼ cup of the olive oil, sprinkle with salt and pepper, and toss the quarters well by hand, making sure to rub and coat each piece in the oil and spices. It's okay if they fall apart a little.

Heat a large cast-iron skillet over medium until hot. Add 1 tablespoon of the olive oil and then the cauliflower to the pan, cut side down. Sear for 2 to 3 minutes, or until deeply caramelized, then gently rotate each piece to its other cut side and sear for another 2 to 3 minutes. Finally, place each quarter on its rounded side and transfer the pan to the oven. Roast for about 15 minutes, or until a small knife pierces the thick stalk easily. Remove from the oven.

To plate up, smear the yogurt sauce across a medium serving dish. Set the large hunks of cauliflower on top of the sauce and spoon the relish over everything. Sprinkle with pomegranate seeds and serve immediately, family-style, with steak knives.

Serves 4 to 6

For the Yogurt-Tahini Sauce

½ cup unsweetened, plain Greek-style coconut yogurt (such as Cocojune Pure Coconut)

¼ cup tahini

1 tablespoon freshly squeezed lemon juice

1 teaspoon ground turmeric

½ teaspoon kosher sea salt

Freshly ground black pepper

For the Cauliflower

1 large head of cauliflower (about 2 pounds), tough outer leaves removed, quartered

¼ cup plus 1 tablespoon extra-virgin olive oil, divided

½ teaspoon kosher sea salt

Freshly ground black pepper

Caper-Currant Relish (page 25)

¼ cup pomegranate seeds

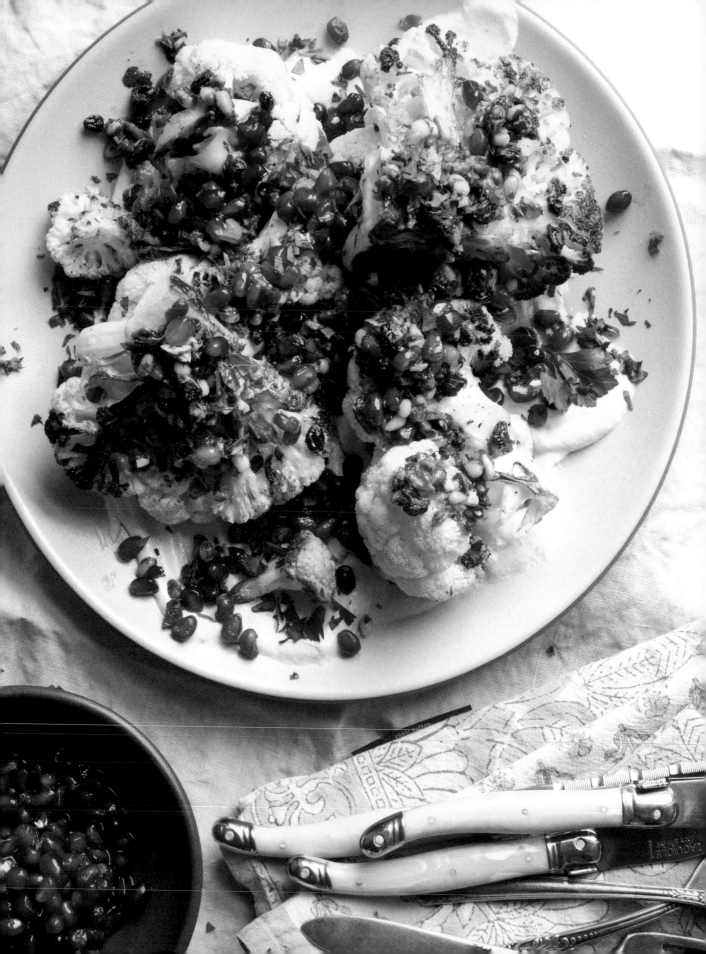

Cauliflower Cannellini Bean Mash

This is my favorite substitute for mashed potatoes. The combination of beans with a touch of cauliflower creates a familiar creamy yet fluffy texture. It's also high in fiber, nutritious, and versatile. You can use it as a dip, served alongside roasted or fried chicken, or as a topping for shepherd's pie. I love it blended with Garlic Confit and lots of fresh black pepper. Yum.

Place the beans and cauliflower in a medium pot, add the water and salt, and bring to a gentle boil over medium-high heat. Simmer on low for about 10 minutes, or until the cauliflower is soft and tender.

Using a slotted spoon, transfer the beans and the cauliflower to a food processor. Add the ghee, Garlic Confit, and pepper, and pulse a few times, until the mixture is thick and resembles a rustic mash. Taste and add more salt if desired. Be careful not to overprocess. Serve warm.

Serves 2 to 4 as a side dish

2 (15-ounce) cans cannellini beans, rinsed and drained

1 cup (about 6 ounces) cauliflower florets

2 cups water

¾ teaspoon kosher sea salt, plus more as needed

2 tablespoons ghee

1 tablespoon Garlic Confit (page 18)

Freshly ground black pepper

Tip
To enrich with a cheesy flavor profile, you can add 1 to 2 tablespoons of nutritional yeast while blending.

Swap It
You can substitute 2½ cups of cooked beans (page 40) for the canned beans.

If you don't have garlic confit on hand, just add 1 clove of fresh garlic to the pot of beans and cauliflower as they cook, and blend it up with everything else.

Garlicky Greens with Apple Cider Vinegar

These are simple and perfectly seasoned garlicky greens. I love the bitter, peppery flavor of broccoli rabe here, but you can switch the rabe out for Broccolini or leafy greens such as kale, collard, mustard greens, or Swiss chard. It's a two-step process done in one pan that ensures a successful outcome. First, season and soften the greens by quickly blanching them in salty boiling water. Then drain them and throw them back into the pot with hot oil, garlic, and a dash of acid.

Bring the water and salt to a boil in a large stockpot.

Add the greens to the water, using tongs to push the ends into the water if necessary, and blanch them for 30 to 60 seconds, until the tough stems are slightly softened. Do not overcook. Transfer to a sieve, rinse quickly with cold water, and drain the water from the pot.

Return the pot to the stove and let it warm over medium-high heat, 1 to 2 minutes. Add the olive oil, then drop the greens back in. It may sizzle and splash a little, so be careful. Let the greens char, about 2 minutes, then add in the garlic and toss everything around to incorporate. Cook for another minute or two, stirring a few times, then add the vinegar and stir once more. Season with a dash of salt and pepper if you like. Transfer to a serving dish immediately.

Serves 2 to 4 as a side dish

2 quarts water

1 tablespoon kosher sea salt, plus more for seasoning

1 bunch of broccoli rabe (about 1 pound), 1 inch of ends trimmed off

2 tablespoons extra-virgin olive oil

1 large clove garlic, minced

1 tablespoon apple cider vinegar

Freshly ground black pepper (optional)

Swap It

You can use the vinegar called for above, or substitute a squeeze of citrus juice or a splash of wine.

Sauce It

To take this up another notch, drizzle the greens with Whole-Lemon Anchovy Dressing (page 9).

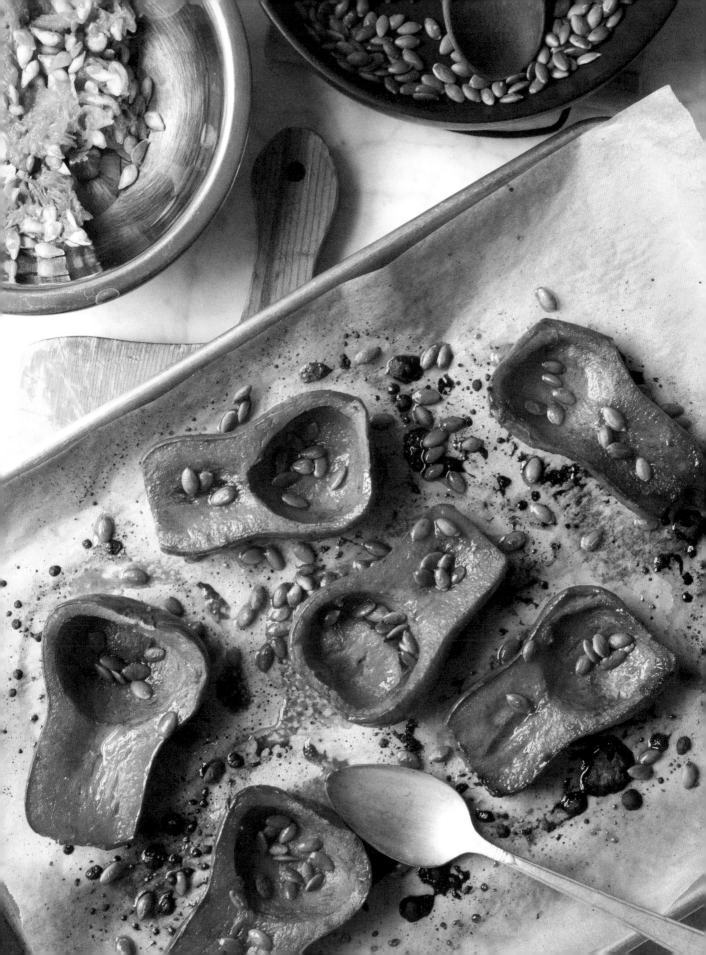

Roasted Honeynut Squash

I first noticed this cute squash varietal at my local market when I lived in Upstate New York in 2016, and had to know where it came from. I did what I do best: I totally nerded out. I learned that honeynut squash was bred specifically for its concentrated flavor and nutrient density as a joint project between Cornell University and chef Dan Barber, co-owner of Blue Hill at Stone Barns in New York. Honeynut squash is sweet and nutty and packs twice the amount of beta-carotene as its cousin, butternut squash. Similar to delicata squash, the skin is thin and tender and can be eaten, so there is no need to peel it before roasting. Roasted with simple seasonings, honeynut squash becomes literally sweet like candy, and looks lovely on a platter sprinkled with Za'atar Toasted Pepitas (page 34).

Serves 4 to 6

1 teaspoon kosher sea salt

½ teaspoon ground cinnamon

4 small honeynut squash

2 tablespoons extra-virgin olive oil, plus more for serving

2 tablespoons maple syrup

¼ cup Za'atar Toasted Pepitas (page 34)

Preheat the oven to 425°F, and line a baking sheet with parchment paper.

Combine the salt and cinnamon in a small bowl and mix.

Cut the hard top ends off the squash, then cut the squash lengthwise. Scoop out and discard the seeds.

Place the squash on the prepared baking sheet in a pile and drizzle with the olive oil and maple syrup. Toss them by hand, making sure to coat the vegetables evenly.

Sprinkle the cinnamon salt over the squash on both sides, making sure they are seasoned evenly. Spread out the vegetables, cut side down.

Roast for about 30 minutes, or until caramelized and fork-tender.

Transfer the squash to a serving dish, drizzle with more olive oil, and sprinkle with the toasted seeds.

Serve immediately, or store in an airtight container in the fridge for up to 3 days.

Wild Mushrooms with Ghee, Herbs + Sherry Vinegar

Mushrooms are the perfect side dish to prepare during the week when you may be short on time or needing to get dinner on the table fast. They cook quickly and absorb all the delicious flavors in the pan, making them plump and juicy. You can use one varietal, or mix and match your favorites. They are earthy and pair well with fresh herbs like thyme, rosemary, and sage and are a rich source of fiber and vitamin D. I love whipping up a quick batch to serve alongside roasted salmon, grilled steak, or simply to spoon over toast.

Heat a large skillet with a lid over medium for about 3 minutes. Add the ghee and mushrooms, simmer, and stir to combine. Cover and let the mushrooms sweat until they release their natural juices, about 3 minutes.

Uncover, add the salt, thyme, vinegar, and lemon juice, and stir to combine. Cook until most of the liquid in the pan has evaporated, 3 to 5 minutes.

Remove from the heat, sprinkle with parsley, and serve immediately, or allow to cool, transfer to an airtight container, and store in the fridge for up to 3 days.

Serves 2 to 4

3 heaping tablespoons ghee

1 pound wild mushrooms (such as chanterelle, morel, shiitake, hen of the woods, or a mixture of mushrooms), wiped clean with a damp cloth

½ teaspoon kosher sea salt

1 teaspoon minced fresh thyme leaves

1 tablespoon sherry vinegar

1 teaspoon freshly squeezed lemon juice

¼ cup chopped fresh flat-leaf parsley, plus more for garnish

Tip
Serve over the Yogurt-Tahini Sauce (page 128).

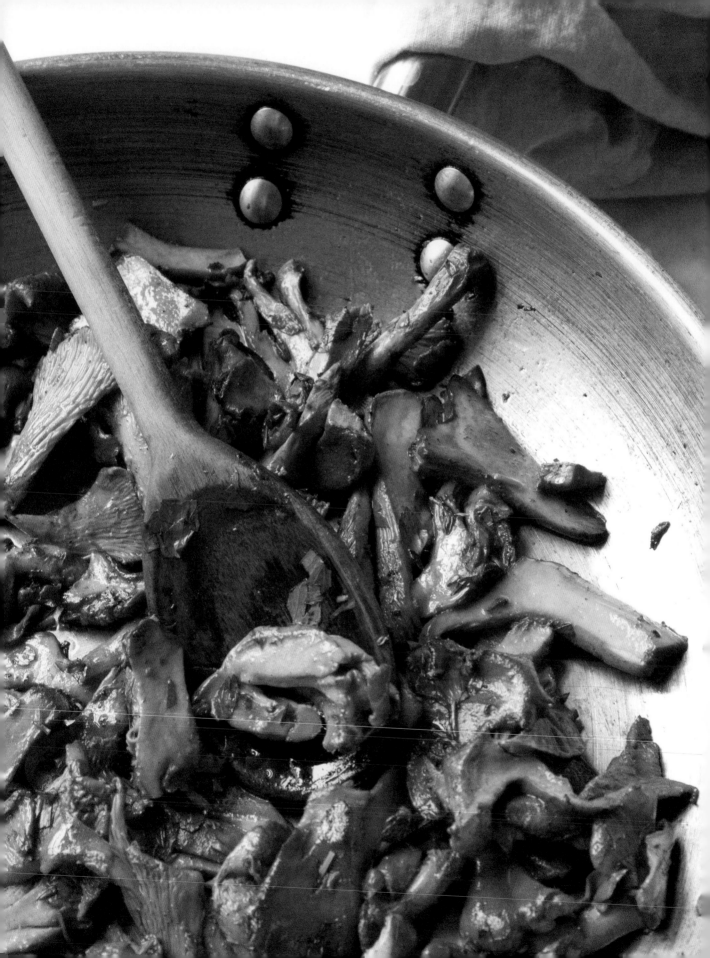

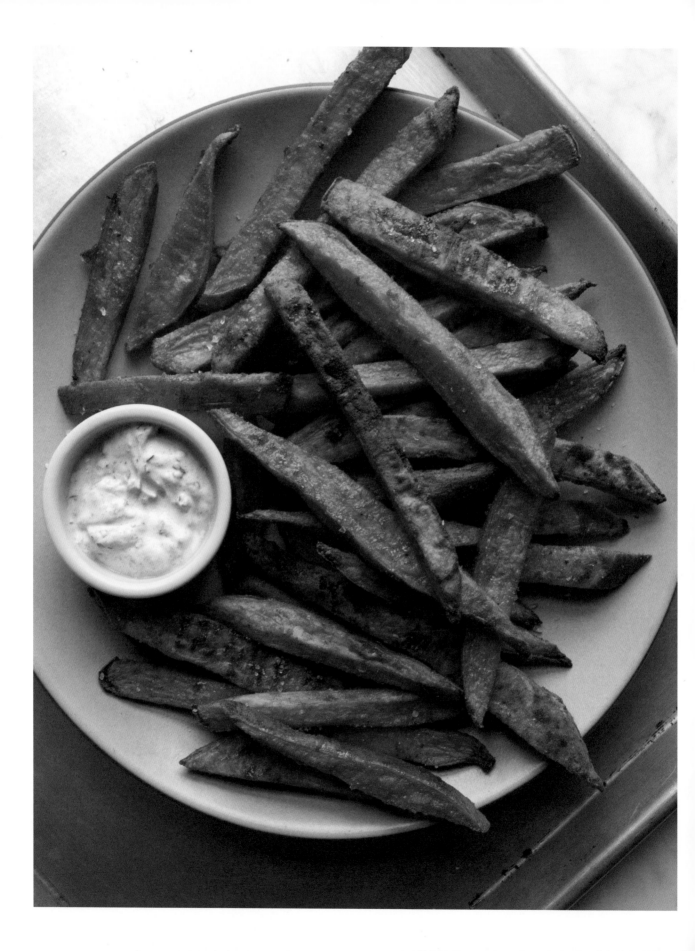

Crispy Oven-Fried Sweet Potatoes

I'm a nerd who loves to research and experiment in my kitchen. I stumbled across this technique and it really brings an upgrade to your oven-fry game. Soaking sweet potatoes in cold water prior to oven-frying will result in delightfully crispy fries at home. This is because soaking helps to release their natural starches, making them more available during cooking. A minimum of 30 minutes will do, but several hours or overnight is even better. Another thing to note is to hold off on the salt until just before serving. Salt brings out moisture in foods, and we are really trying to keep these dry and crispy in the oven while roasting. Lastly, these will develop their final stages of crunchiness while cooling, so do your best not to pick at them until they are ready!

Serves 2 to 4 as a side dish

1½ pounds small sweet potatoes, cut into ¼-inch strips

1 teaspoon garlic granules

1 teaspoon ground paprika

1 teaspoon coconut sugar

3 tablespoons extra-virgin olive oil

1 teaspoon kosher sea salt, plus more for serving

Tip
Serve with Chipotle Aioli (page 21) or Coconut Yogurt Tzatziki (page 31).

Begin by soaking the sweet potatoes in a large bowl of cold water for a minimum of 30 minutes or overnight, refrigerated.

When you're ready to make the fries, preheat the oven to 450°F and line 2 baking sheets with parchment paper.

In a small bowl, mix the garlic, paprika, and coconut sugar.

Drain and rinse the sweet potatoes and pat *very* dry with a dish towel or paper towels. Rinse out and dry the bowl and place the fries back in. Drizzle with the olive oil and sprinkle the spice mixture over, tossing the sweet potatoes by hand and making sure to coat well with the spices.

Spread out the potatoes evenly in a single layer on the baking sheets, making sure they aren't touching each other.

Roast for 15 minutes, then remove from the oven and flip each fry with tongs. Rotate the pans and return to the oven for another 15 to 20 minutes, or until the fries are crispy and dark golden brown.

Remove from the oven and allow to cool for 10 minutes, so they can crisp up even more.

Sprinkle with salt and serve immediately.

Span-ish Frittata
with Spinach

This is a mash-up of two classics: a traditional Spanish tortilla and an Italian frittata. A tortilla is an omelet made with potatoes, onions, and eggs that gets inverted onto a plate and then returned to the pan and stove top to finish cooking and is served at room temperature. A frittata is an Italian omelet that is essentially a crustless quiche that can be filled with all sorts of meats, vegetables, and cheeses. It begins on the stove and gets transferred to the oven to finish cooking. Here I've used the classic Spanish tortilla ingredients of potatoes, onions, and eggs, but I've added some fresh spinach and skipped the whole plate-inversion step by finishing it in the oven.

Preheat the oven to 375°F.

Heat a large cast-iron or nonstick skillet on medium, then add the olive oil and 1 teaspoon of the salt.

When the oil is hot, using a large spoon, carefully place all the potatoes and onions in the pan. Gently spread the vegetables into an even layer. (Don't worry, they will cook down and submerge eventually.) Cook for about 10 minutes, or until the potatoes and onions soften and become slightly golden, stirring occasionally.

In a large bowl, whisk the eggs, the remaining ½ teaspoon of salt, and some pepper to blend. When the vegetables are cooked, use a slotted spoon and transfer them to the egg mixture. Add the spinach and fold everything together using a rubber spatula.

Drain the oil from the pan, leaving about 1 tablespoon, and allow the drained oil to cool completely for another use.

Reheat the skillet over medium and return the egg mixture to the pan. Allow the eggs to set for 2 to 3 minutes, undisturbed, until a crust forms, then transfer the skillet to the oven. Bake for 25 to 30 minutes, until puffed up and golden.

Remove from the oven and allow to cool completely. Slice like a pie and serve at room temperature, or transfer to an airtight container and store in the fridge for up to 3 days.

1 cup extra-virgin olive oil

1½ teaspoons kosher sea salt, divided

3 medium-size Yukon gold potatoes (about 1 pound), peeled and cut into 1-inch cubes

1 yellow onion, thinly sliced

8 large eggs

Freshly ground black pepper

2 handfuls of baby spinach

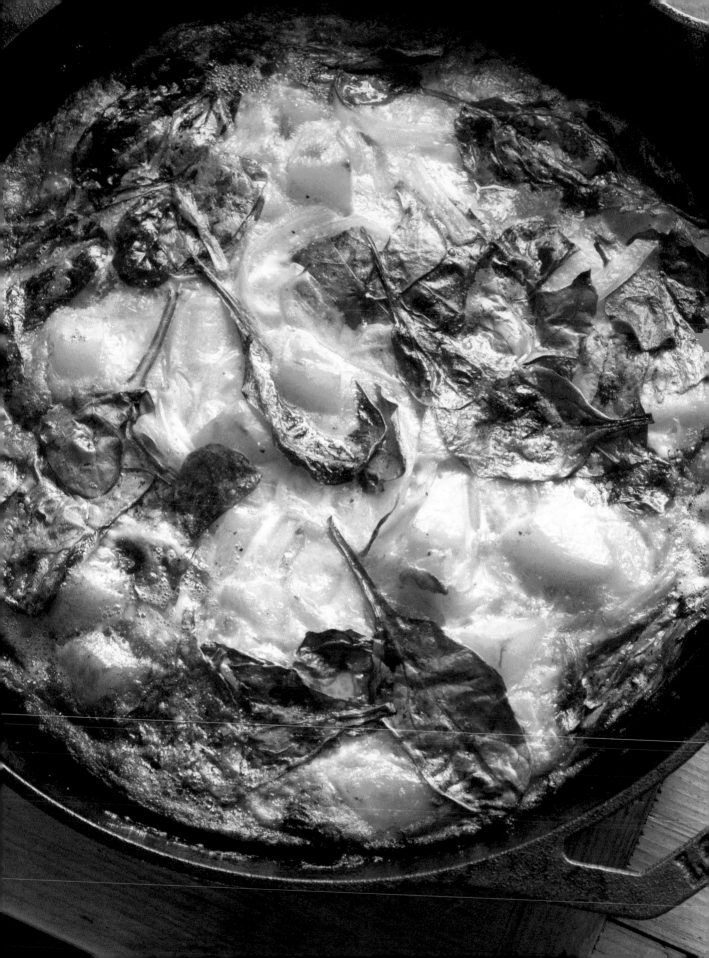

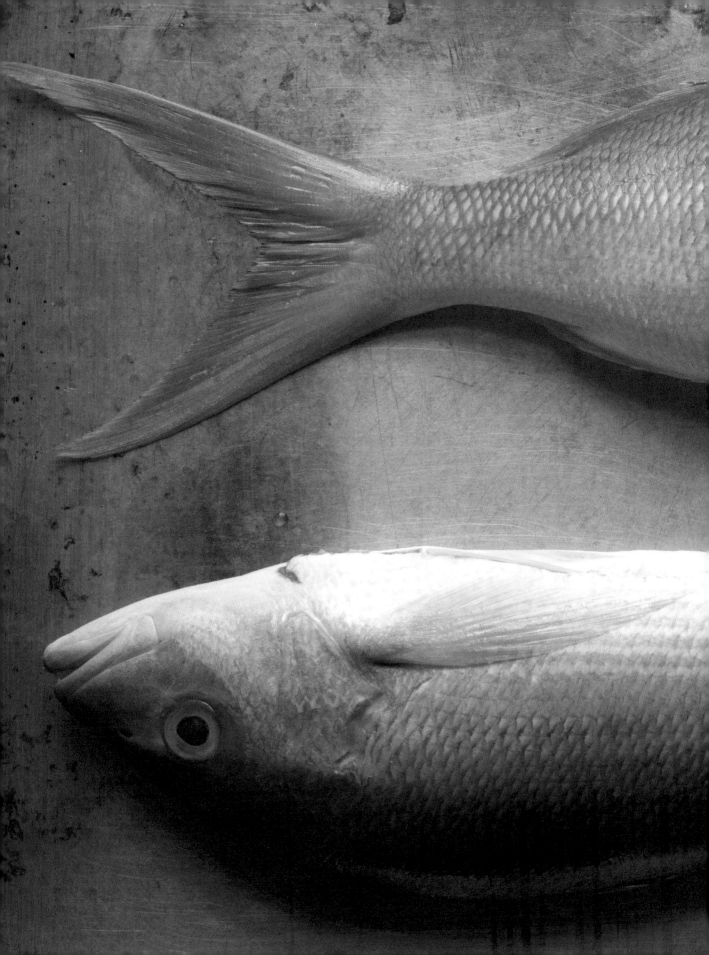

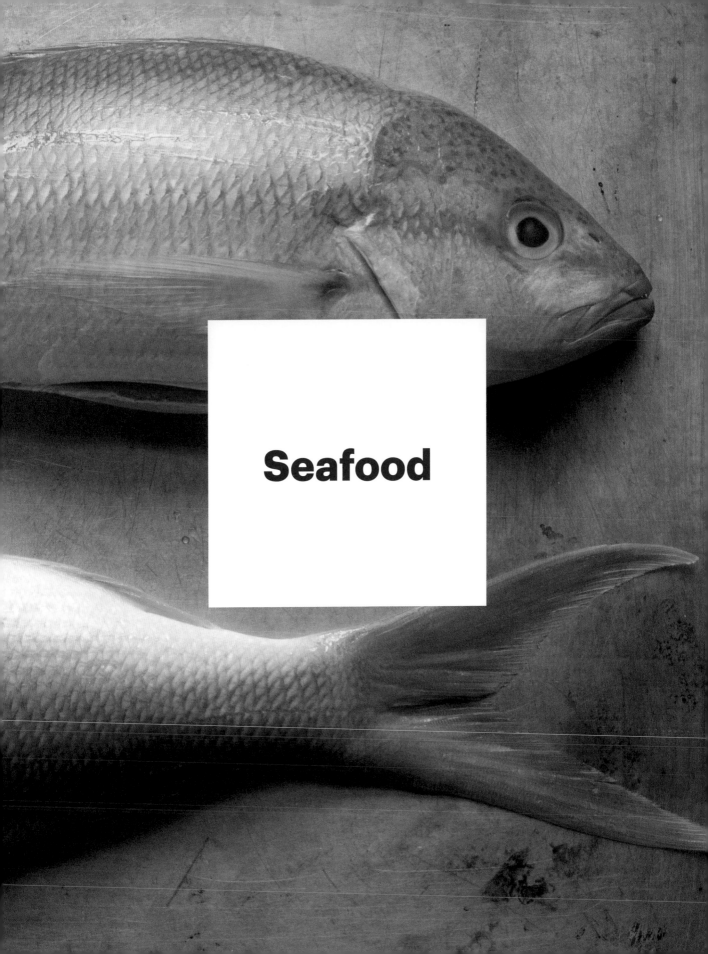

Seafood

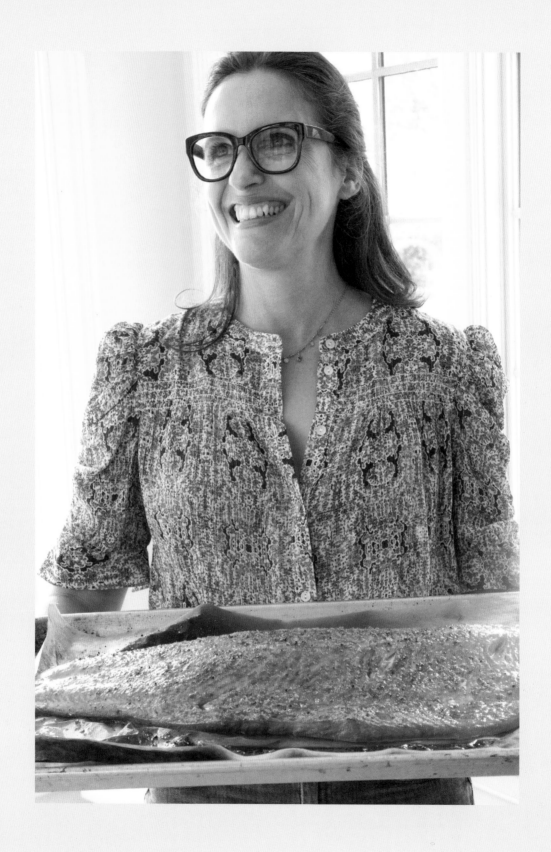

Blow Their Socks Off

I got lucky the first time I had a real dinner party. I read a recipe in a magazine that had a simple preparation: roast the salmon at 500 degrees for 15 minutes with a little olive oil, salt, and pepper. That's it. A fatty piece of fish in a screaming-hot oven with a little seasoning. It was perfection. I couldn't believe how easy it was, and my guests devoured it.

This was a light-bulb moment for me as a home cook. The only two things I needed to do were find the best piece of fish possible and cook it properly. I have held on to the same principle since then; beautiful, simple ingredients often don't need much. Your job is to hunt them down, learn the best way to prepare them so they shine, and get out of the way! The dishes that impress people the most are often the easiest to make. It's okay to splurge on good ingredients for special meals because they do all the work for you.

For years, salmon was the only thing I made when we had dinner parties. I have since moved from roasting to broiling my salmon because I prefer the crunchy exterior you get from broiling. The next time you decide to have a dinner party, try making Crispy Broiled King Salmon (page 148). Pick a sauce like the House Chimichurri (page 5), and set them both out on your countertop to let your guests serve themselves. You will blow their socks off. There will be no leftovers.

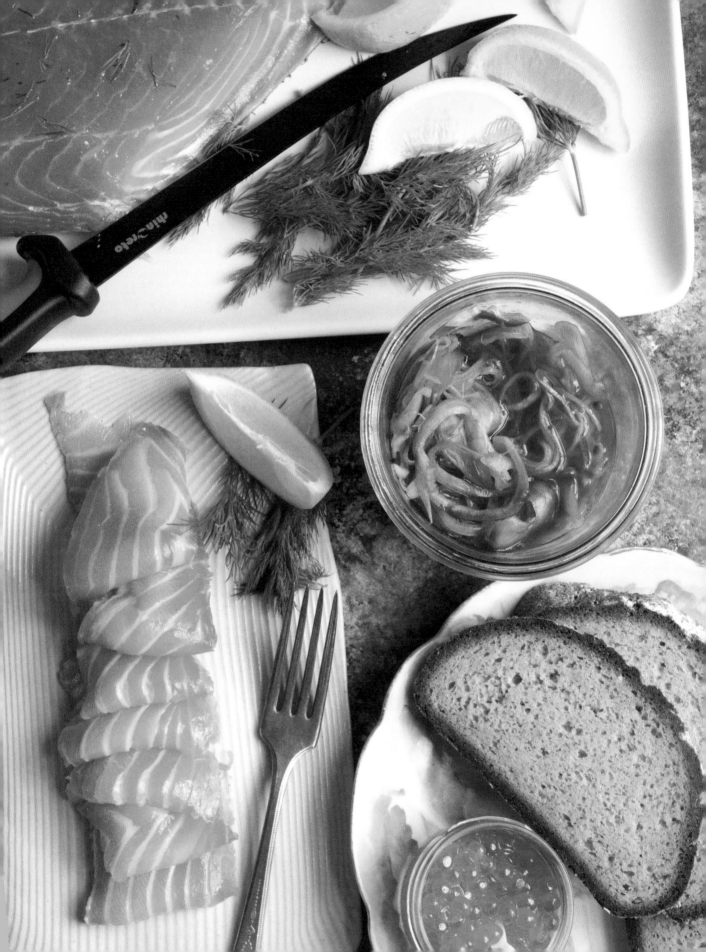

Citrus-Cured Lox

The first apartment I lived in by myself in New York City after college had an incredible deli a block away that delivered, at all hours (of course), the most outrageously fresh, doughy, warm bagels. They came with a fat slab of cream cheese and a giant mound of the most luscious lox I had ever had in my life. My friends and I used to order these bad boys at 1:00 a.m. I don't eat bagels with cream cheese anymore, and I'm in bed by 10:00 p.m. these days, but I still love lox, and once you discover how easy this is to make, you may never buy store-bought cured salmon again. Make sure to use kosher salt and stick with the suggested prep time, as different kinds of salts and curing times will yield varied results that might not be so desirable. If you're wondering about the sugar content, most of it gets rinsed off after curing. This recipe will deliver a medium cure of silky, luscious fish that will melt in your mouth. I like to start the (mostly hands-off) 24-hour process on Friday morning so that when I wake up on Saturday morning, we have gorgeous lox for the whole weekend. Great for when we have company, too! It's wonderful bagel-style atop slices of Grain-Free Vegan Boule (page 201). I like to serve it with salmon roe, pickled red onion, dill, and slices of lemon.

You can ask your fishmonger to remove the salmon's pin bones, or do it yourself using a small pair of tweezers.

Line a large rimmed baking sheet with a large piece of foil.

In a medium bowl, combine the salt, sugar, zests, and dill and mix them thoroughly by hand.

Spread half the curing mixture in the center of the foil, then place the fish on it skin side down. Cover the salmon with the remaining mixture, making sure to spread it evenly so the fish is completely covered. Bring the edges of the foil up and over the filet, crimping it in the center to completely enclose the fish in a tight bundle.

Place another baking sheet on top of the fish, and weight it with several large cans or a heavy pot. Place in the fridge for 24 hours, flipping the fish halfway through the process.

Recipe continues

Serves 8

1 cup kosher sea salt

1 cup coconut sugar

1 tablespoon finely grated lemon zest (from 1 large lemon)

1 tablespoon finely grated lime zest (from 2 small limes)

1 tablespoon finely grated orange zest (from 1 medium orange)

½ cup chopped fresh dill

1 (2-pound) wild king salmon fillet, skin on, pin bones removed

Once the curing is complete, remove the salmon from the foil and rinse it under cold water to remove the curing mixture, then pat dry with paper towels. On a cutting board, place the salmon skin side down and slice as much salmon as you want thinly on the diagonal with your sharpest, longest knife until you reach the skin. Cut the salmon slices away from the skin and transfer to a serving dish. For clean cutting, use a wet towel to wipe down the blade in between slices, if necessary.

Wrap up tightly any unsliced leftovers in plastic wrap and store in the fridge for up to 3 days.

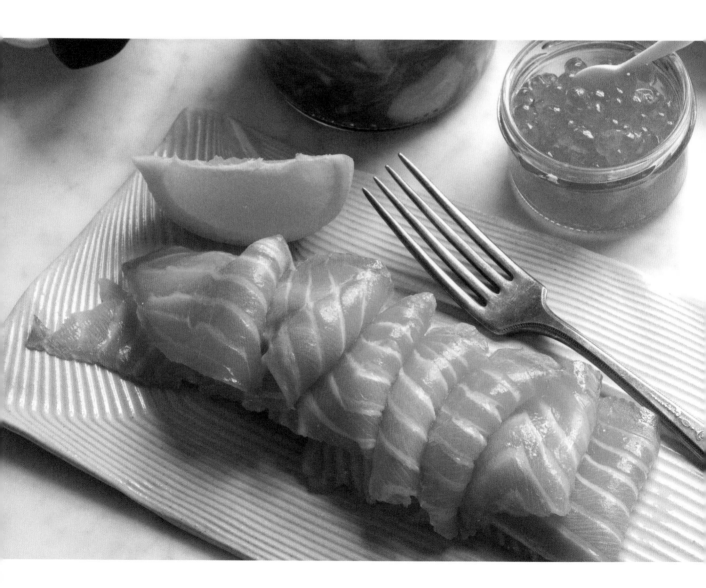

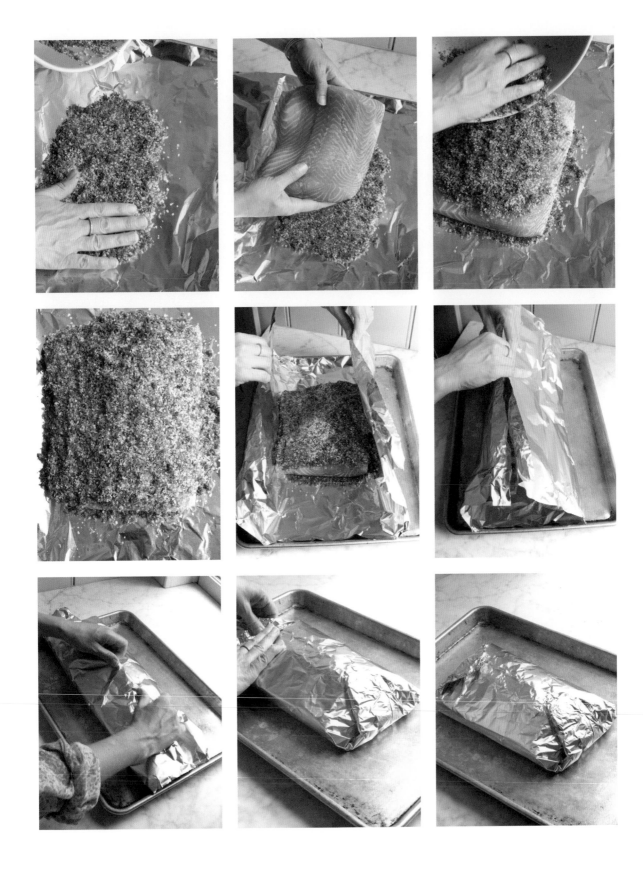

Crispy Broiled King Salmon

If you'd like to blow the socks off your people, I suggest you give this a shot. It's worth mentioning that the key here is to try and find the FRESHEST piece of salmon you can. You're looking for lush, buttery flesh. Ideally you have a broiler in your oven that will crisp up all the fat in the salmon to create a gorgeous crunchy exterior, but if not, crank your oven to 500 degrees and roast it instead. This method can get smoky, so get your exhaust fan going or open the windows if you have to. The parchment paper might burn during cooking; that's okay—don't chicken out, this is good! That's the price to pay for restaurant-style fish!

Preheat the oven broiler to high, and adjust the rack to about 8 inches below the heating element. If you don't have a broiler, preheat the oven to 500°F. Line a rimmed baking sheet with parchment paper.

Place the salmon skin side down on the baking sheet. Drizzle and rub 3 tablespoons of the olive oil over the fish and season it evenly with salt. Broil or roast for 12 to 15 minutes, or until it is dark, crispy, and bubbling at the edges.

While the salmon cooks, heat a small nonstick skillet over medium-high, then add 1 teaspoon of the olive oil. When the oil is shimmering hot, add the lemon halves cut sides down and char for 1 to 2 minutes, until fragrant and blackened. Transfer to a small plate.

Remove the fish from the oven carefully and allow to rest for 10 minutes. I like to serve it straight from the pan, but you can transfer it to a serving platter if you prefer. If you decide to transfer it to a serving dish, you can lift it up from the paper by slipping 2 spatulas underneath. Serve with the grilled lemons.

Serves 4

1½ pounds skin-on king salmon (1½ to 1¾ inches thick)

3 tablespoons plus 1 teaspoon extra-virgin olive oil

1 teaspoon kosher sea salt

2 lemons, halved

Freshly ground black pepper (optional)

Sauce It
Try the Green Onion Salsa (page 6), House Chimichurri (page 5), Cherry Tomato Confit (page 18), or Caper-Currant Relish (page 25).

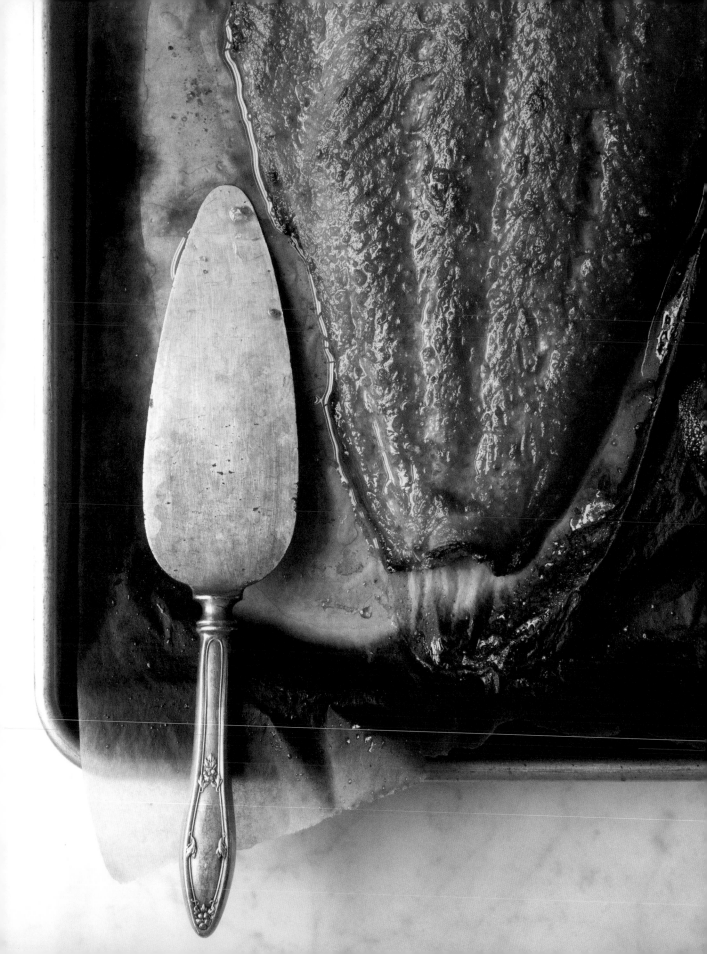

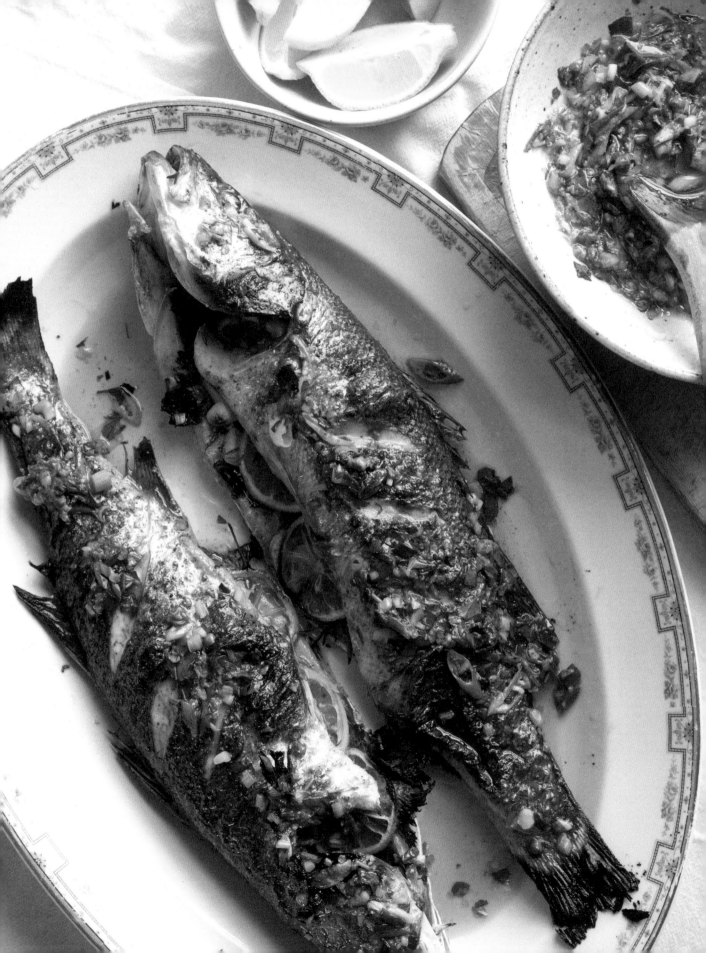

Whole Roasted Branzino

As always with fish, the key to success is making sure you get the freshest fish possible. Ask your local fishmonger when they get their whole-fish delivery and see if you can order ahead of time. It makes a huge difference. Roasting a whole fish does two things: first, bones impart tons of flavor to the meat, and second, the skin seals in the moisture, keeping things nice and juicy. The delicate and slightly sweet flesh of branzino lends itself beautifully to these bright fresh flavors. This preparation is super easy, and the presentation is stunning. You can serve this at a casual summer party or for Christmas Eve dinner (see Tips). This gets messy on the table, so I like to set out some extra bowls for everyone to throw their bones into while they make their way through the meal.

Preheat the oven to 450°F, and arrange a rack about 8 inches from the upper heating unit. Line a baking sheet with parchment paper.

Rinse the fish with cold water and pat very dry with paper towels, inside and out. Use a sharp knife to gently score 3 diagonal lines, about 1 inch apart and ⅛ inch deep, into the flesh on one side of the fish. Place the fish on the baking sheet.

In a small bowl, combine the salt, cumin, and paprika. Slice 1 lemon into thin rounds.

Drizzle and rub 2 to 3 tablespoons of olive oil over the fish on both sides and inside the cavity. Season the fish with the spice mixture on both sides and inside the cavity. Make sure the scored side of the fish is facing up, divide the herbs into 2 bundles, and stuff them inside each cavity. Place some garlic slices over the herbs, top with 3 lemon slices, and drizzle with a little more olive oil.

Roast the fish for 20 minutes, then broil on the highest setting for 2 minutes, or until the skin is very crispy and browned.

Remove from the oven and let rest for 10 minutes. Transfer to a serving dish and drizzle with more olive oil. Serve with the other lemon cut into quarters.

Serves 2

- 2 gutted, descaled whole branzino, each 1 to 1½ pounds
- 2 teaspoons kosher sea salt
- ½ teaspoon ground cumin
- ½ teaspoon ground paprika
- 2 lemons, divided
- Extra-virgin olive oil, as needed
- 1 handful of fresh herbs (such as a combination of parsley and dill), stems trimmed and divided
- 1 large clove garlic, thinly sliced and divided

Sauce It
Serve with the Green Onion Salsa (page 6), Caper-Currant Relish (page 25), or House Chimichurri (page 5).

Swap It
Substitute sea bass or red snapper for the branzino.

Tips
Serve with sticky white rice, Garlicky Greens with Apple Cider Vinegar (page 131), or Steak Knife Roasted Vegetables (page 122).

Double or triple the recipe for larger dinner parties by simply spreading the fish out between 2 baking sheets and broiling a sheet at a time at the end. Easy!

Seared Scallops with Garlic Ghee

We love visiting the northern tip of Long Beach Island, on the Jersey Shore. There's a small town called Barnegat Light, near Viking Village, a fishing enclave. Besides being a lovely and charming place with an interesting history, the area also happens to be home to one of the three major scalloping ports in New Jersey. We frequent a fish shop in Viking Village, right at the dock. The boats go out every morning and return with fresh seafood every day, including the most sweet and succulent scallops I've ever had. They inspired me to keep this preparation simple and to celebrate their inherent tenderness and sweetness. The most important part of this recipe is to try and find the best scallops you can. Make friends with your local fishmonger and get tips on when the fresh seafood deliveries arrive, so you get first pick.

Lay the scallops out on a large plate, pat them dry on both sides with paper towels, and season with salt and pepper on both sides.

Heat a medium skillet on medium-high for about 4 minutes, or until smoking hot. Add the olive oil, then add half the scallops, spreading them out so they don't touch. Sear for 2 to 3 minutes, until nicely charred, then flip and finish cooking for another minute. Transfer them to a serving plate and repeat with the remaining scallops, loosely covering the first batch with foil to keep warm.

Once all the scallops are cooked, reduce the heat to medium-low, and add the ghee and garlic. Cook for 1 minute, or until the garlic is fragrant but still hasn't taken on much color, then add the lemon juice. Scrape all the brown bits from the pan, creating a rich, concentrated pan sauce. Add 1 tablespoon of the parsley and stir to combine.

Spoon the sauce over the scallops, and finish with the remaining parsley. Serve immediately.

Serves 2 to 4

1 pound scallops (18 to 20)

¾ teaspoon kosher sea salt

Freshly ground black pepper

1 tablespoon extra-virgin olive oil

3 tablespoons ghee

2 large cloves garlic, minced

1 to 2 tablespoons freshly squeezed lemon juice

2 tablespoons chopped fresh flat-leaf parsley, divided

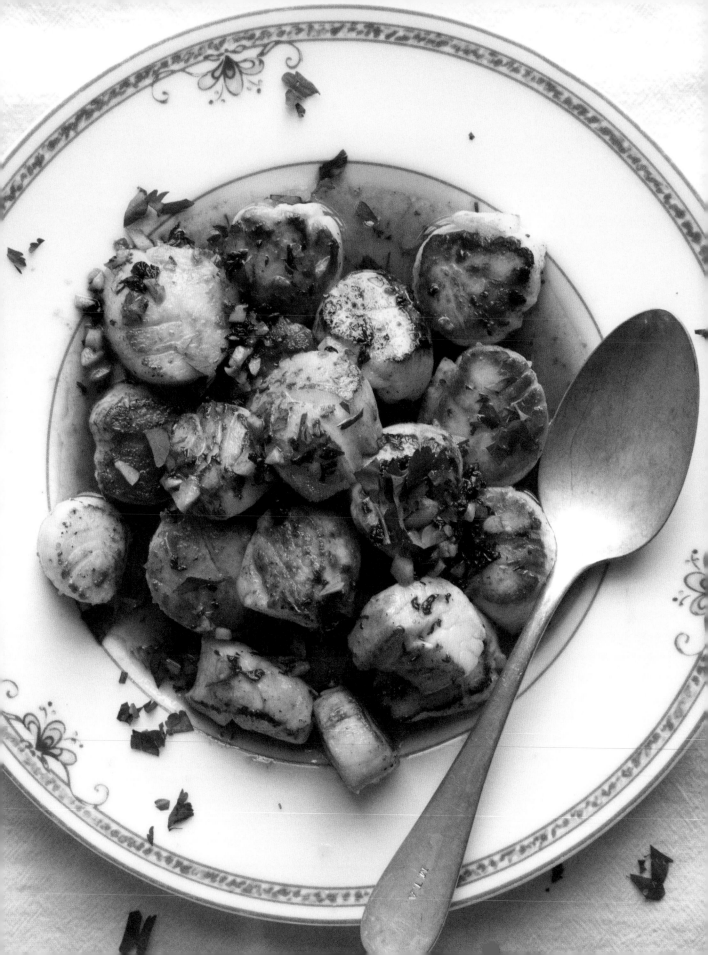

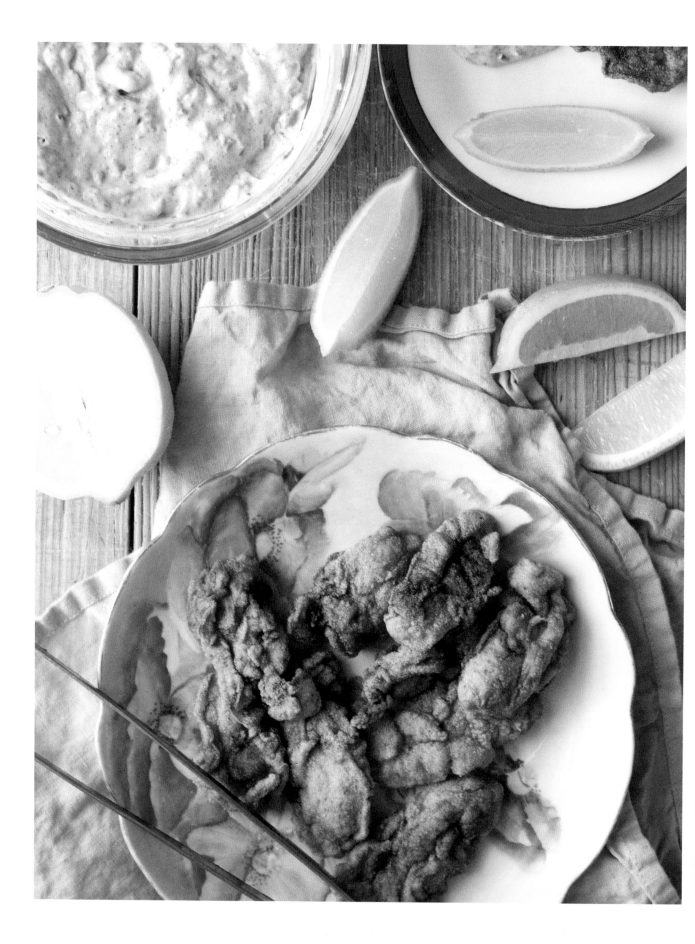

Fried Oysters with Remoulade Sauce

It may delight you to know that a jar of shucked oysters is surprisingly inexpensive, and they tend to be extra plump and juicy, making them perfect for frying. I've dusted these in a blend of cassava and tapioca flours, which fries up light and crunchy, and paired them with my creamy and tart remoulade sauce. To ensure that your oysters don't turn out greasy, make sure to try and keep the frying oil at 350°F. Also, remember to be careful when frying anything in your kitchen and watch out for the occasional oil spurt jumping from the pan.

First, make the remoulade by placing all the ingredients in a medium bowl and mixing until well combined. Cover and place in the fridge for a minimum of 2 hours to allow the flavors to develop. You can also prepare this a day ahead if you like.

Empty the jar of oysters into a sieve and rinse carefully with cold water. Drain them, then transfer to a plate lined with paper towels and pat dry. Once the paper towels have soaked up the excess water, discard them, leaving the moist oysters on the plate.

In a wide, shallow bowl, mix the tapioca and cassava flours, baking powder, and all of the spices. Season with salt and pepper.

Heat the avocado oil in a medium Dutch oven over medium (it should reach 2 or 3 inches up the side of the pan), until it reaches 350°F on an instant-read thermometer, 8 to 10 minutes.

Line a plate with paper towels.

Working in batches of 4 oysters, dredge each oyster in the flour mixture. Using tongs, carefully add the 4 prepared oysters to the pan. Try to keep the oil at 350°F by adjusting the heat as necessary. Cook them until golden brown on the underside, about 2 minutes, then gently flip and cook for another minute. Using a slotted spoon, carefully remove them from the oil and transfer to the paper towel–lined plate.

Continue this process until all the oysters are fried. Transfer all the oysters to a serving dish, and serve immediately with the remoulade sauce and lemon wedges on the side.

Serves 4 to 6 as an appetizer

For the Remoulade

1 cup avocado-oil mayonnaise (such as Follow Your Heart Avocado Oil Vegenaise)

¼ cup finely minced shallots

2 tablespoons minced chives

1 heaping tablespoon sweet relish

1 tablespoon freshly squeezed lemon juice

1 heaping tablespoon country-style Dijon mustard

1 tablespoon minced capers

2 cloves garlic, finely chopped

1 teaspoon gluten-free Worcestershire sauce

1 teaspoon ground paprika

¼ teaspoon Kosher sea salt

Freshly ground black pepper (optional)

For the Oysters

1 (16-ounce) jar shucked oysters

¼ cup tapioca flour

¼ cup cassava flour (such as from Otto's or Bob's Red Mill)

½ teaspoon baking powder

1 teaspoon granulated onion

1 teaspoon granulated garlic

½ teaspoon ground paprika

Kosher sea salt

Freshly ground black pepper

1 quart avocado oil

1 lemon, cut into wedges

Wild Fried Fish Tacos with Quick Pickled Slaw + Chipotle Aioli

I really love tacos. *All* tacos. But maybe fried fish tacos are the best of all. Besides being a healthy option, they are crispy, creamy, salty, spicy, and sometimes sweet, and can be loaded with a variety of flavors and textures. The batter in this recipe is light and extra crunchy thanks to sparkling water. The pickled cabbage slaw is bright and tangy, and the Chipotle Aioli (page 21) is perfectly sweet and smoky. All the elements here come together like a dream. If you decide to make the pickled slaw, homemade tortillas, and the aioli all together, be sure to set aside more time and luxuriate in the process. Otherwise, if you'd like to break it up, I would suggest making the aioli, the slaw, and the tortilla dough a day ahead.

Make the slaw first: In a sieve set over a bowl, toss the cabbage with the salt and let it sit for 20 minutes to release excess liquid and drain. In another small bowl, toss the red onions with just enough vinegar to cover and let macerate while the cabbage drains, about 15 minutes.

When the cabbage has drained, transfer to a medium bowl and add the onions, without the vinegar. Add the cilantro, lime juice, and olive oil, and mix everything well. Taste and adjust seasoning to your liking.

For the fish, mix the tapioca flour with a pinch of salt in a shallow medium bowl. In a separate medium bowl, whisk together the cassava flour with 1 teaspoon of the salt, all the spices, and the sparkling water to make a batter.

Heat the avocado oil in a medium Dutch oven over medium (it should reach 2 or 3 inches up the side of the pan) until it reaches 350°F on an instant-read thermometer, 8 to 10 minutes.

Serves 4

For the Quick Pickled Slaw

3 cups finely shredded purple cabbage

1 teaspoon kosher sea salt

½ cup thinly sliced red onion (from about a quarter of an onion)

Red wine vinegar

¼ cup roughly chopped cilantro

1 tablespoon freshly squeezed lime juice

2 tablespoons extra-virgin olive oil

For the Tacos

¼ cup tapioca flour

1 teaspoon kosher sea salt, plus more for seasoning

½ cup cassava flour (such as from Otto's)

1 teaspoon paprika

½ teaspoon ground cumin

½ teaspoon garlic granules

1 cup sparkling water

1 quart avocado oil

1½ pounds firm, white-fleshed wild fish (such as halibut, cod, or pollock), cut into 8 equal pieces

8 Cassava Tortillas (page 197) or Sweet Potato Tortillas (page 197)

Chipotle Aioli (page 21)

2 limes, quartered

Working in batches, dredge 4 pieces of fish in the tapioca flour, then drop them into the bowl of batter, making sure to toss and coat thoroughly. Carefully transfer each piece to the pan, one by one, and fry, making sure not to overcrowd the pan, 3 to 4 minutes per side, until golden brown on both sides.

Using a spider strainer or large slotted spoon, transfer the fried fish from the pot to a rack set over a baking sheet or a paper towel–lined plate. Repeat with the remaining 4 pieces of fish.

Place each piece of fish in a tortilla, top with the pickled slaw, and drizzle with the Chipotle Aioli. Serve with cut lime wedges.

Swap It

Substitute cabbage leaves for the tortillas for a lighter taco. Substitute a coconut-lime crema (Swap It on page 31) for the Chipotle Aioli if you're avoiding nightshades.

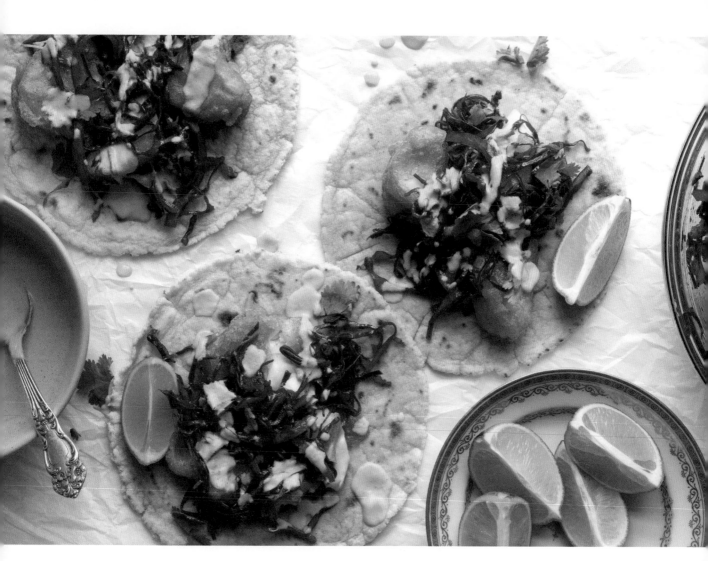

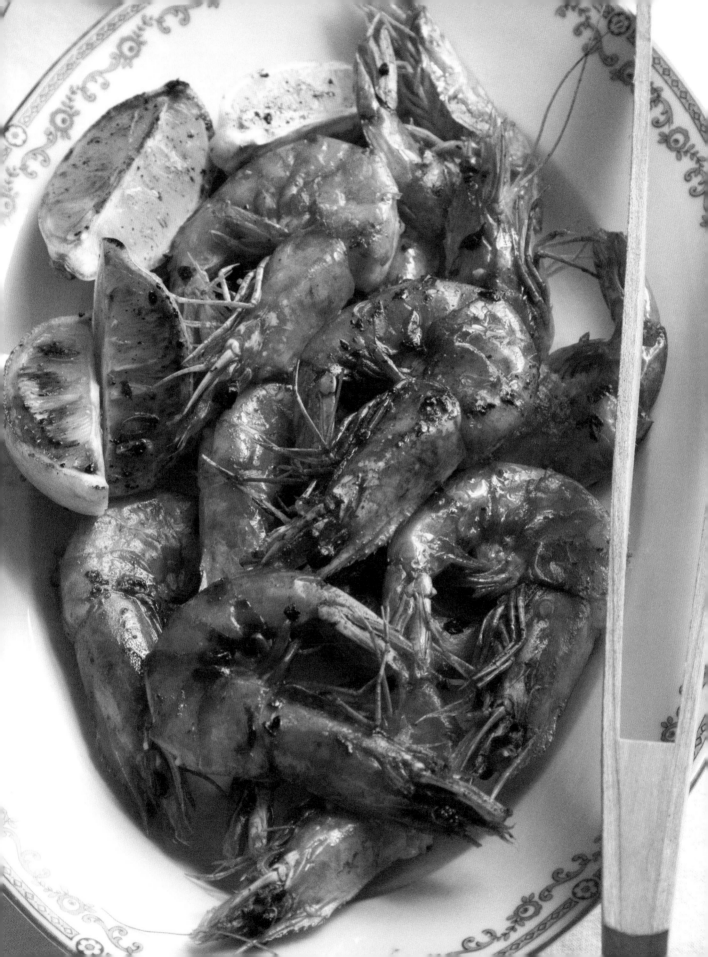

Whole Garlic Prawns with Charred Lemon

To me this is hands down the best way to eat prawns. Leaving the shell on prawns protects the delicate flesh from overcooking and traps all their juicy flavors inside, making them succulent and absolutely delicious! Plus, there is a magic that happens when you combine shellfish with garlic, ghee, and lemon. You must eat them with your hands, and you must be prepared to suck on their heads and legs without fear! If you've never tried it, you're in for a treat. I can polish off an entire platter on my own.

If you'd like to double the recipe, use two skillets.

Clean the prawns first: Using a small paring knife, carefully cut through the shells of all the prawns along the outer back curve of each shrimp, cutting through the shell itself and about ⅛ inch into the flesh the entire way from the head to the tail, and rinse out the veins underneath with cold water. Make sure to leave the shells, heads, and tails intact. Pat very dry and place in a medium bowl.

Add the garlic, olive oil, and salt, toss to combine, and refrigerate for 1 hour, uncovered.

About 30 minutes before you're ready to cook the prawns, take them out of the fridge and let them come to room temperature.

Heat a large cast-iron skillet over medium-high until screaming hot, about 5 minutes.

Add 1 tablespoon of the ghee, wait for it to ripple in the pan, then carefully add half the prawns in a single layer. Cook undisturbed for about 3 minutes, or until deeply browned underneath, then use tongs to flip the shrimp and cook for another 30 seconds. Transfer to a serving plate. Add the other tablespoon of ghee and repeat until all the prawns are cooked, making sure not to overcrowd the pan. Allow to rest for 5 to 10 minutes.

Keep the pan on and add the lemon quarters, cut side down. Char until deeply browned on one side, about 1 minute. Transfer the lemons to the serving plate with the prawns, sprinkle with fresh parsley, and serve.

Serves 2

1 pound fresh large prawns, head and shell on

4 large cloves garlic, minced

1 tablespoon extra-virgin olive oil

1 teaspoon kosher sea salt

2 teaspoons ghee, divided

1 lemon, quartered

1 tablespoon roughly chopped fresh Italian parsley

Swap It
Substitute olive oil for the ghee if you prefer.

Flounder Meunière

This is a simplified version of the traditional French dish sole meunière. I used to work at a French restaurant in New York City, and we prepared this classic dish bone-in and deboned it tableside. It was quite a presentation. The dish typically uses a combination of clarified butter and browned regular butter. To make this easier, I'm using boneless fillets, and I've omitted the butter to keep it virtually dairy-free—and replaced it with ghee, which is inherently nutty and "brown" in flavor (see Building an Alternative Pantry on page xiv). I've also swapped cassava flour for regular flour, and the result is so close to the real thing: delightfully light and crispy, with bright citrus and a toasty, buttery pan sauce.

Place the flour in a wide, shallow bowl. Season the fillets on both sides with salt and pepper, and dredge them each in the flour. Set them aside on a plate until you are ready to cook.

Heat a large nonstick skillet over medium-high for 3 to 4 minutes. Add 3 tablespoons of the ghee. When it moves around like water in the pan, add 2 fillets. Cook for 3 to 4 minutes, until crisp and golden underneath, then carefully flip using a fish spatula. Cook for another minute, then transfer to a serving dish and cover loosely with foil.

Add the remaining ghee and repeat the process with the remaining fish. Once you have finished cooking the fish, spoon the excess ghee in the pan over the fillets and sprinkle with the fresh parsley.

Serve immediately with fresh lemon wedges.

Serves 2 to 4

½ cup cassava flour (such as from Otto's or Bob's Red Mill)

4 (4- to 6-ounce) flounder fillets

Kosher sea salt

Freshly ground black pepper

6 tablespoons ghee, divided

1 to 2 tablespoons chopped fresh flat-leaf parsley

1 lemon, quartered

Swap It
You can easily substitute sole for the flounder.

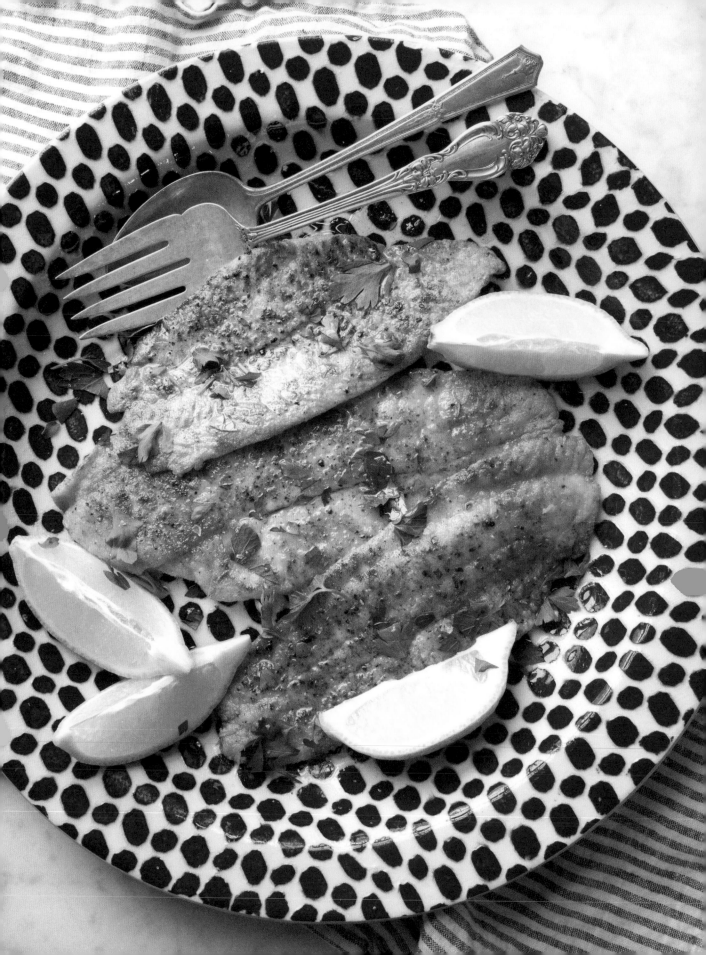

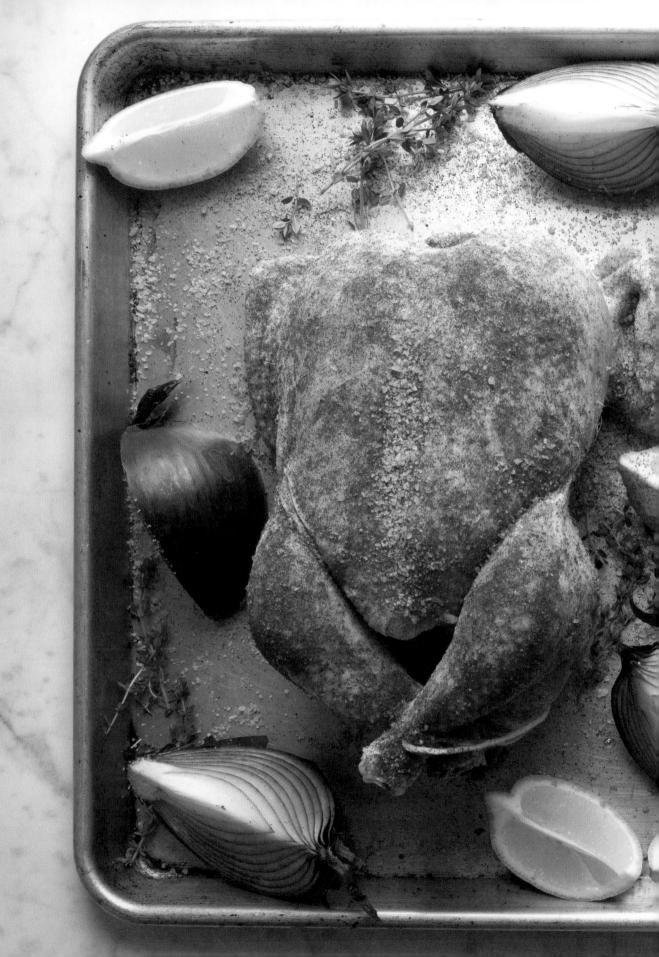

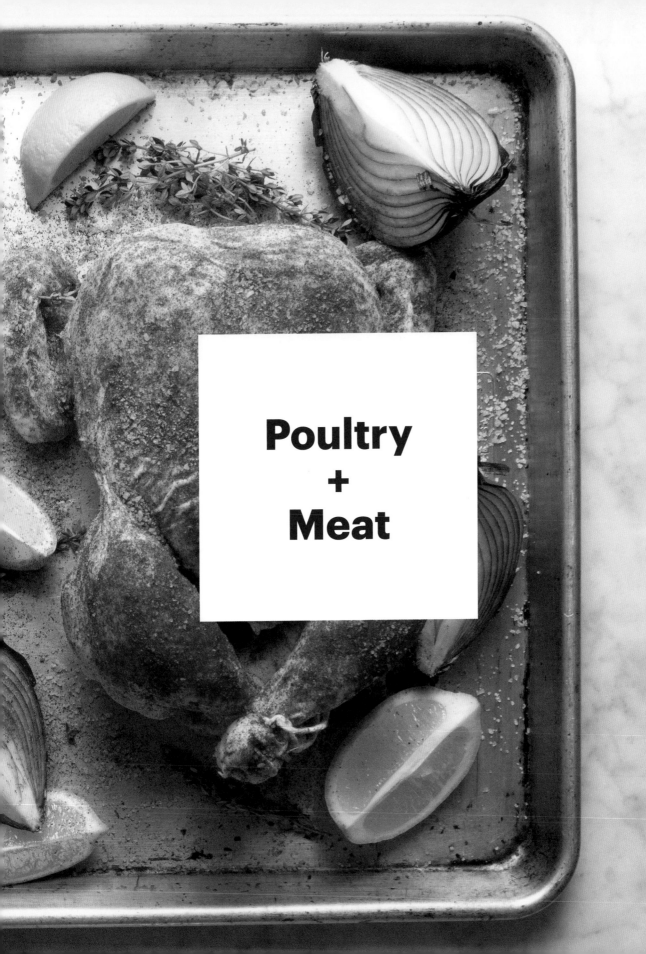

Poultry
+
Meat

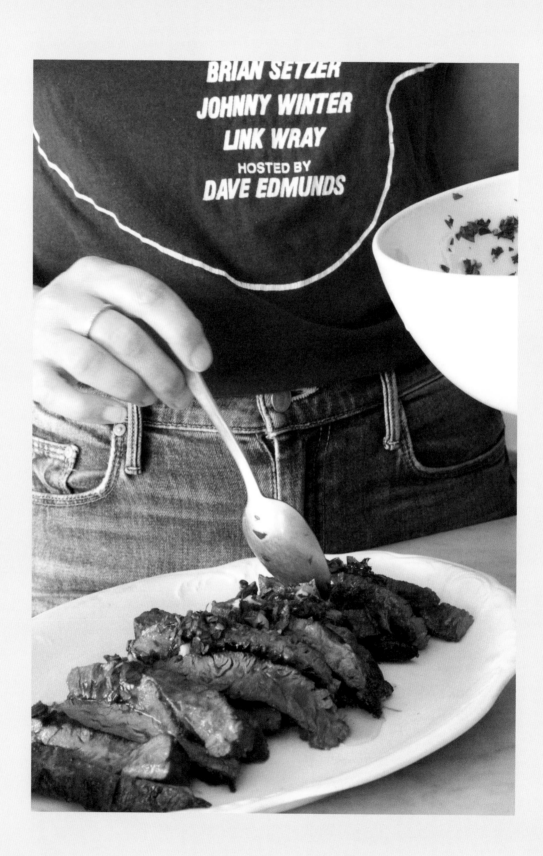

Making Choices at the Meat Counter

When it comes to meat and poultry, I have only a few important things to say: First, I prefer to eat darker cuts of poultry (on the bone, if possible) because I find them more flavorful and juicier. I like crispy skin, too, and I'm willing to fight for it! I prefer steaks on the rarer side of things and stewed meat to be fall-apart tender. But these are all personal preferences—things I like certain ways on my own plate. You can eat all the chicken breasts and well-done steak you want, if that's what you like. But the most important choice I make about meat (and one I encourage you to investigate, if you haven't already) is my commitment to supporting regenerative agriculture.

There are so many incredible humans out there doing the important work of regenerative agriculture, which focuses on restoring and rebuilding the soil we use to grow plants and raise animals. This is very different to industrial agriculture, which is the large-scale production of animals and crops that involves the use of routine antibiotics and growth hormones in animals and chemicals on crops. Using humane animal management practices makes meat that's better for the environment and for our communities. A regenerative approach fosters a thriving, living ecosystem that improves soil health, reduces water pollution, and cultivates biodiversity. It also creates a resilient natural system that doesn't require chemical intervention to manage diseases or pests. The fat content in the meat of these animals is lower, the brain-boosting omega-3 and omega-6 fatty acids are higher, and they contain more antioxidant vitamins. The earth and our bodies are better for it. Even if you are vegan, it's important for all of us to be aware of the differences between industrialized agriculture and regenerative agriculture.

At the store, look for meat that's labeled "grass-fed" and "pastured," and do some quick research to find out how the producer raises its animals. If you can't find these products at your local market, you can go online, as many regenerative farms and ranches ship all over the country.

Gochujang Wings

The only thing I like about the Super Bowl is that it provides a halftime show and an excuse to hide in the kitchen and make a ton of chicken wings. The key to getting juicy, crispy wings without frying them is to air-dry them in the fridge overnight, uncovered, after a coating of salt, coconut sugar, and baking powder. This requires a little extra prep, but it's a mostly hands-off process that ensures extra crispiness and juiciness. Gochujang is a thick sweet and spicy Korean chili paste that can be found in most grocery stores. (Not all brands are gluten-free, so make sure to check the label.) This delicious sauce pairs perfectly with fatty, crispy chicken wings, making this the ultimate game-day dish—or any-day-of-the-week dish!

If you are avoiding nightshades, try using the Sticky Plum BBQ Sauce (page 26) instead.

Line a large baking sheet with parchment paper, and place a rack over it.

Wash and then pat the wings very dry with paper towels. Place them in a large bowl.

In a small bowl, mix the salt, baking powder, and sugar. Add the mixture to the wings and toss by hand to coat everything. Transfer the wings to the rack, making sure they are spread out evenly and not touching each other, and place them in the fridge, uncovered, for about 24 hours.

When you're ready to cook the wings, remove them from the fridge and allow to reach room temperature for about 30 minutes. Preheat the oven to 350°F.

Transfer the wings to a plate, brush the rack with olive oil, and return the wings to the rack, again making sure they don't touch. Bake for 20 minutes, until golden brown.

Serves 4 to 6

2 pounds chicken wingettes (or drumettes, or full wings)

2 teaspoons kosher sea salt

2 teaspoons aluminum-free baking powder

1 tablespoon coconut sugar

Extra-virgin olive oil, as needed

2 tablespoons ghee

2 cloves garlic, minced

1 tablespoon minced ginger (from a roughly 1-inch piece)

¼ cup gluten-free gochujang

3 tablespoons maple syrup

1 tablespoon apple cider vinegar

1 tablespoon freshly squeezed lime juice

⅓ cup thinly sliced green onions, for serving

Lime wedges, for serving

While the wings roast, heat a small saucepan over medium. Add the ghee, garlic, and ginger, reduce heat to medium-low, and cook until fragrant, about 1 minute. Add the gochujang, maple syrup, vinegar, and lime juice. Whisk together and simmer until thick and bubbling, about 2 minutes.

Remove the wings from the oven and transfer to a large mixing bowl. Pour the gochujang sauce over them, and use a rubber spatula to toss until coated evenly. Remove the rack from the baking sheet. Return the wings and all the sauce to the parchment paper on the baking sheet and bake the wings for another 15 minutes.

Remove from the oven again, flip using tongs, and return to the oven. Broil on high on the center rack for 2 to 3 minutes, until the wings are crispy and deeply caramelized.

Remove finally from the oven and let rest for 10 minutes. Serve straight from the pan or on a serving platter, scattered with green onions and lime wedges.

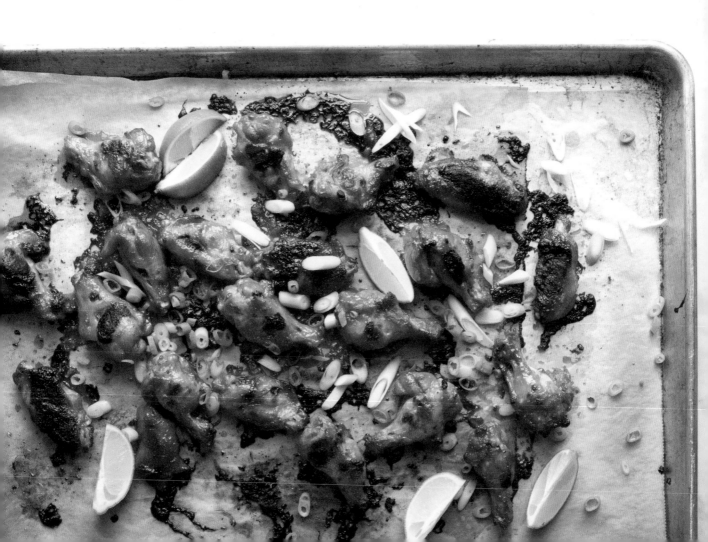

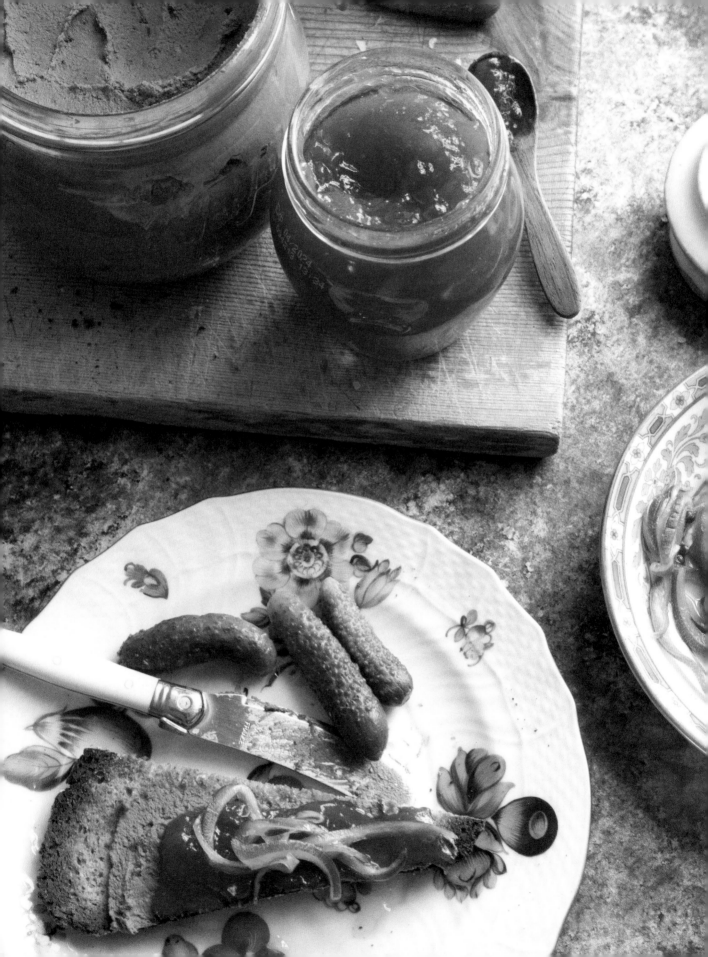

Chicken Liver Pâté

Every recipe in this book serves an aspect of your health in some intentional way. Chicken liver contains more iron than beef liver, so if you are anemic, this might help build your iron back up more effectively. I realize that liver is not for everyone, but I encourage you to give this a try if you are on the fence. It's blended with lots of aromatics, herbs, and ghee, making it very palatable, rich, and decadent. Perfect for special occasions *and* perfect for supportive nourishment!

Heat a large skillet over medium for about 3 minutes. Add 4 tablespoons of the ghee and reduce heat to medium-low, then add the shallots and sauté until soft and translucent, 4 to 5 minutes. Add the garlic and cook for 1 minute, just until softened. Add the livers, thyme, whiskey, and salt, and cook until the alcohol has evaporated and the livers are browned but still pink inside, 5 to 6 minutes.

Transfer everything in the pan to the bowl of a food processor, add the nutmeg and the remaining 4 tablespoons of ghee, and process until smooth and creamy, 30 to 60 seconds. Salt to taste.

Transfer the pâté to a glass bowl or pint-size jar and allow to cool. Cover the pâté directly with plastic wrap, pressing down on the surface to create an airtight seal, then close the jar. Store in the fridge for up to 5 days.

Bring to room temperature for about 30 minutes before serving with your choice of accoutrements.

Serves 4 to 6

8 tablespoons ghee, divided

½ cup finely chopped shallot (from 2 to 3 large shallots)

2 large cloves garlic

1 pound organic chicken livers

2 teaspoons fresh thyme leaves

3 tablespoons whiskey

Kosher sea salt

¼ teaspoon ground nutmeg

Your choice of toast points, sliced cucumbers, sliced apples, Quick Pickled Red Onions (page 28), apricot jam, and/or cornichons, for serving

"Sour Cream" + Onion Chicken Thigh Schnitzel with Chip Crumbs

Shouldn't we all have a killer schnitzel recipe in our allergen-friendly arsenal? This is a gussied-up version of giant chicken fingers that's really geared toward adults, although I guarantee that even the most skeptical youngster will devour these without batting a lash. To make them grain-free, I ditched the bread crumbs altogether and ground up a few bags of my favorite lime plantain chips. Because I'm not a fan of white meat, I went straight for juicy chicken thighs instead. I left out the egg wash and replaced that with tangy yogurt, which worked perfectly for tenderizing and dredging the cutlets, and added a classic sour cream and onion twist. Oh boy. The results were beyond my wildest dreams. If you can't find the brand of chips I suggest here, just go for plain salted plantain, cassava, or potato chips. Serve these with loads of fresh lemon wedges and the Butter Lettuce with Fresh Herbs, Toasted Maple Sunflower Seeds + Marlit's Vinaigrette (page 70), or Lemon Spaghetti (page 109), and watch them disappear.

Rinse and pat the chicken thighs very dry with paper towels and transfer to a baking dish. In a small bowl, mix the salt with the spices and season both sides of the thighs. Add the yogurt and toss by hand, making sure to coat the chicken evenly. Cover with plastic wrap and refrigerate for a minimum of 2 hours, or overnight.

Empty the lime chips into the bowl of a food processor, and pulse until they resemble coarse bread crumbs, about 60 seconds. Transfer the crumbs to a wide, shallow bowl.

Line a baking sheet with parchment paper. Line a second baking sheet with a wire rack, or a large plate with paper towels. One by one, coat and press each thigh into the plantain crumbs and place on the prepared baking sheet.

Heat a large skillet to medium-high for about 4 minutes. Add the tablespoons of ghee and oil. When the oil moves around like water in the pan, using a fork to stab one end, add 2 to 3 schnitzel to the pan. Don't overcrowd the pan. Reduce the heat to medium and fry

Serves 4 to 6

8 organic boneless, skinless chicken thighs

1 teaspoon kosher sea salt

½ teaspoon granulated garlic

½ teaspoon granulated onion

½ cup unsweetened, plain Greek-style coconut yogurt (such as Cocojune Pure Coconut)

2 (5-ounce) bags Barnana Acapulco Lime plantain chips

3 heaping tablespoons ghee, plus more if needed

3 tablespoons avocado oil, plus more if needed

2 lemons, cut into wedges, for serving

until deep golden brown, 3 to 4 minutes, then flip. Cook for another 3 minutes, or until deep golden brown on the second side. Transfer to the rack or paper towels to drain. Repeat until all the schnitzel are cooked, adding an extra tablespoon of ghee and oil along the way if necessary. There should be a thin layer of fat in the pan at all times.

Serve with fresh lemon wedges.

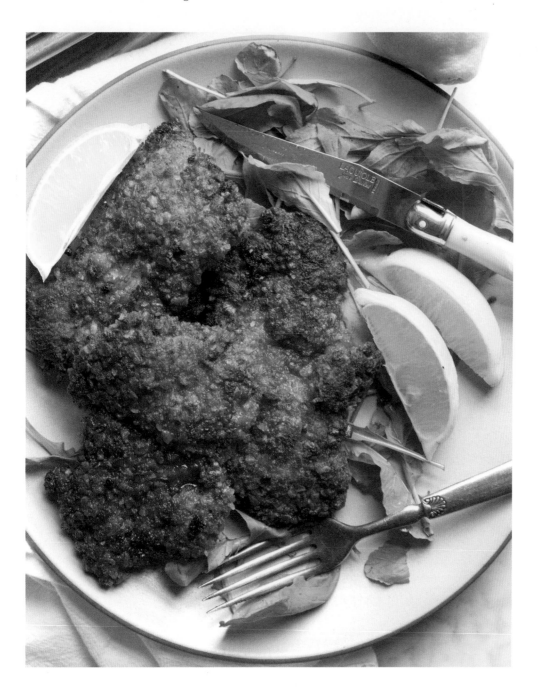

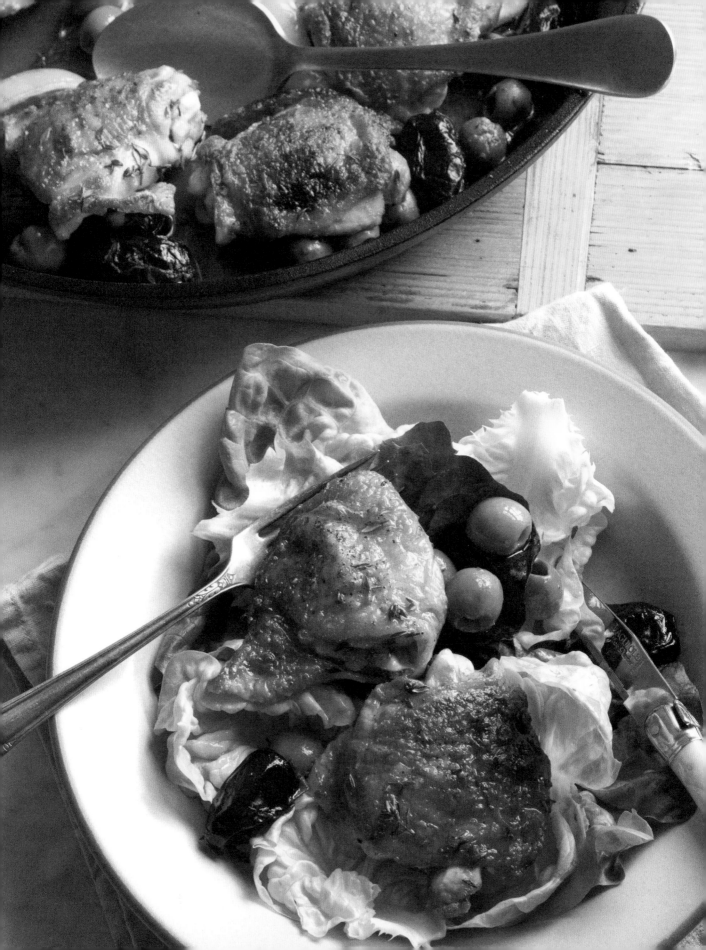

Chicken Thighs with Green Olives, Dates, Lemon + Butter Lettuce

This is one of the most delectable recipes in this book. The magic here is the extra pan drippings. Once the chicken has fully cooked, you are left with heavenly crispy thighs and an abundance of a concentrated schmaltzy, lemony, buttery pan sauce studded with caramelized dates and roasted olives that you will drizzle over a bed of tender lettuce leaves. It is the perfect plate.

Preheat the oven to 375°F.

Wash the chicken and pat very dry with paper towels. Place the chicken thighs in a large dish or on a cutting board and season with salt and pepper on both sides.

Heat an extra-large cast-iron or ovenproof skillet (at least 12 inches in diameter) over medium-high. Add 1 tablespoon of the ghee, swirl it around, and when little wisps of smoke come off the pan, add the chicken thighs skin side down. Reduce the heat to medium and cook undisturbed until the skin is golden brown and crisp, 12 to 15 minutes, fitting the lemons into the pan cut side down after the first 8 minutes.

Flip the chicken and lemon quarters over, then add the olives, dates, thyme, and remaining 3 tablespoons of ghee, and drizzle everything with the olive oil. Transfer the pan to the oven and roast for 10 minutes.

Remove the chicken from the oven, and gently crush the lemons with a large spoon to release their juices. Tilt the pan and baste the chicken with the pan juices. Return to the oven and cook for another 5 minutes.

Remove from the oven again and allow to rest for 5 minutes. To serve, take a large handful of lettuce and make a bed in a pasta bowl or wide dish. Place 1 to 2 chicken thighs on top, along with some dates and olives, and then spoon the pan juices over everything.

Serves 4 to 6

- 6 bone-in, skin-on chicken thighs (2½ to 3 pounds)
- 1½ teaspoons kosher sea salt
- Freshly ground black pepper
- 4 tablespoons ghee, divided
- 1 large lemon, quartered
- 1 cup pitted green olives, drained
- 12 Medjool dates, pitted
- 6 sprigs of fresh thyme leaves
- ¼ cup extra-virgin olive oil
- 1 head of butter, Boston, or Bibb lettuce, washed, dried, and torn into large pieces

Swap It
Substitute butter for the ghee if you prefer. To make this dairy-free, omit the ghee and butter altogether and use olive oil instead. (For my take on ghee, see page xiv.) You can also substitute any pitted olives you like for the green olives.

Overnight Roast Chicken

Does the world really need another roast chicken recipe? Yes. Yes, it does. But I hope this serves as more of a reminder than a recipe: Remember that when you nail it, roast chicken can be one of the most delicious things you have ever eaten, with all that intense concentrated flavor and schmaltz that collects at the bottom of the pan. It has you standing over the stove hours later, scraping and sopping up any leftover juices you can salvage when you're supposed to be doing the dishes.

Mix the salt and paprika in a small bowl.

Remove any giblets and pull out the fat at the cavity opening of the chicken and discard. Wash and dry the chicken very well with paper towels, inside and out. Place the bird in a roasting dish, rub the spices all over inside and out, and put it in the fridge, uncovered, for 24 to 48 hours.

Bring the chicken to room temperature for an hour prior to roasting. Preheat the oven to 350°F.

Scatter the lemons and onions around the chicken, tuck the wing tips back, tuck the herbs inside the cavity, tie the legs together, and drizzle the ghee all over the bird. Roast for about 45 minutes.

Remove the pan and baste the chicken: First, tilt the pan so the juices run out of the bird. Use a large spoon to crush the lemons, so more juice is released from them, too. This will help create more of a pan sauce. Use this sauce to baste the chicken, then return the pan to the oven. Roast another 45 minutes, basting a few more times during the last half of cooking.

When you can wiggle a leg and it moves easily in the joint (that means the bird has come up to about 165°F in the thickest part of the thigh), the bird is done. Take it out of the oven and let rest for 20 minutes. Carve the chicken into pieces, then return them to the pan and toss the chicken pieces in the pan juices. Serve immediately, straight from the pan, with the onions and lemons.

Serves 4

3½ teaspoons kosher sea salt

1 teaspoon ground paprika

1 (3½-pound) organic whole chicken

1 lemon, quartered

1 onion, peeled and quartered

A few sprigs of fresh thyme

3 tablespoons melted ghee or extra-virgin olive oil

Tip
Freeze the carcass in an airtight container or plastic bag. When you've accumulated a few of them, throw them into a pot with some aromatics and make a simple chicken stock. Add any other leftover veggies that are about to turn. This is a great way to empty the fridge and avoid wasting food.

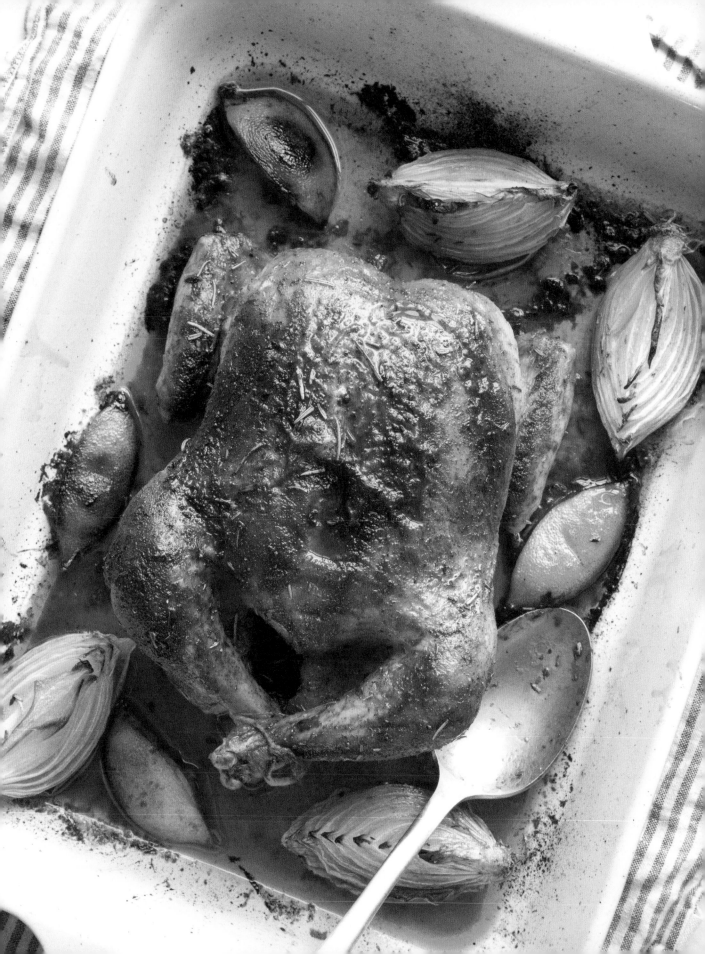

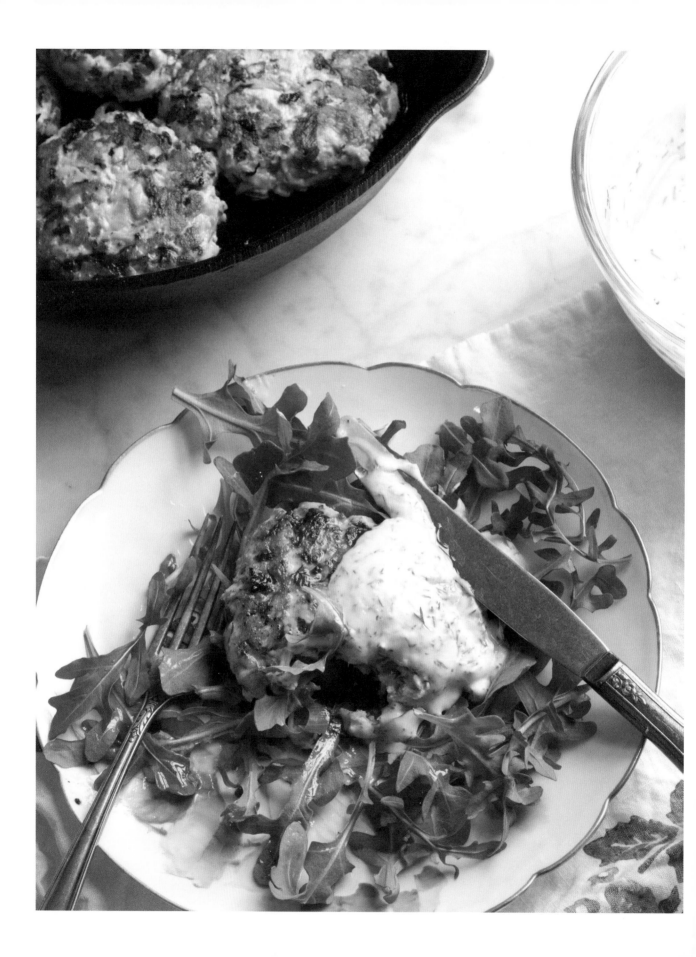

Turkey Zucchini Patties with Coconut Yogurt Tzatziki

These juicy meat-and-vegetable patties are breakfast, lunch, or dinner for me, depending on the day. In general, I find turkey patties to be dry. It's a lean bird, and most recipes use breast meat. I prefer dark meat when it comes to poultry because it contains more fat and therefore more flavor and moisture. Here I'm using ground dark meat, and I've added grated zucchini along with tons of fresh herbs and spices for an extra juicy, flavorful patty that's full of vegetables, too. Throw them over a salad of arugula with sliced radishes and cucumbers, or top off a rice bowl with roasted veggies. This is a great dish to make ahead and reheat, so you can double the recipe and have backup meals ready all week long.

Start the patties: Begin by grating the zucchini into a colander set inside a bowl. Add 1 teaspoon of the salt and mix. Let the zucchini release excess juices and drain for 15 minutes. Squeeze and press out any remaining liquid by hand, and transfer the grated zucchini to a large mixing bowl.

Make the patties: Add the turkey, parsley, green onions, garlic, yogurt, remaining ½ teaspoon of salt, and spices to the zucchini. Mix with a fork until well blended.

Heat a large nonstick skillet over medium, and add 1 tablespoon of oil. Using about ½ cup of the mixture per patty, form 3 turkey patties and set them gently into the hot pan. (The mixture is very wet, so form the patties as you go. Start with 3 patties if your pan can hold them, but don't overcrowd.) Cook the patties for about 5 minutes per side, allowing them to firm up and brown completely before flipping. Repeat with the remaining mixture, adding more oil as needed, transferring the cooked patties to a serving dish. Serve with the tzatziki.

Allow any uneaten patties to cool completely, then transfer to an airtight container and refrigerate for up to 5 days. Reheat patties in the microwave or a small nonstick skillet over medium heat.

Makes 6 patties

For the Patties

1 medium zucchini

1 teaspoon plus ½ teaspoon kosher sea salt, divided

1 pound organic dark-meat ground turkey

½ cup chopped flat-leaf parsley (from 1 small bunch)

3 green onions, chopped

2 large cloves garlic, minced

2 heaping tablespoons unsweetened, plain Greek-style coconut yogurt (such as Cocojune Pure Coconut)

½ teaspoon ground cumin

½ teaspoon ground coriander

Olive or avocado oil, for frying

Coconut Yogurt Tzatziki (page 31)

Middle Eastern Spiced Ground Bison

Inspired by a humble Middle Eastern dish called *hashweh*, warmly spiced beef typically served over rice, this recipe is SO simple and deeply flavorful. It makes for a cozy weeknight dinner for two when served over the Cauliflower Cannellini Bean Mash (page 130), with a light salad and homemade Flatbreads (page 194) on the side. But truth be told, in our house, it never makes it to the dinner table. I usually just make the bison and load it onto the mash when I have time during the day, and as we're milling about before dinner, the four of us snack on it as a heavy appetizer, scooping the flatbreads into it the same way you would with pita and hummus. The bison mixture itself is very flexible; for example, you can change the flavor profile by adding fresh ginger, fish sauce, and coconut aminos in place of the spices listed and serve it over rice.

We love it sprinkled with chopped fresh dill, toasted pine nuts, and pomegranate seeds.

Heat a large skillet over medium; when hot, add the ghee and onions and sauté until soft and slightly golden brown, about 5 minutes. Add the garlic and cook for another minute.

Add the ground bison, salt, and all the spices and mix well. Cook until the meat is browned, stirring occasionally, 8 to 10 minutes.

Stir in the tomato paste and beef stock to combine. Continue cooking until all the liquid has evaporated, about 5 minutes.

Serve immediately, drizzled with olive oil and topped with the dill, pine nuts, and pomegranate seeds.

Serves 2 to 4

1 tablespoon ghee or extra-virgin olive oil

1 medium red onion, diced

2 cloves garlic, minced

1 pound ground bison

¾ teaspoon kosher sea salt

½ teaspoon ground cinnamon

½ teaspoon ground cumin

½ teaspoon ground coriander

¼ teaspoon ground or freshly grated nutmeg

Freshly ground black pepper

1 tablespoon tomato paste

¼ cup low-sodium beef stock or bone broth

Extra-virgin olive oil, for drizzling

Chopped fresh dill, toasted pine nuts (see Tip on page 25), and pomegranate seeds, for topping

Swap It
You can substitute grass-fed ground beef for the bison.

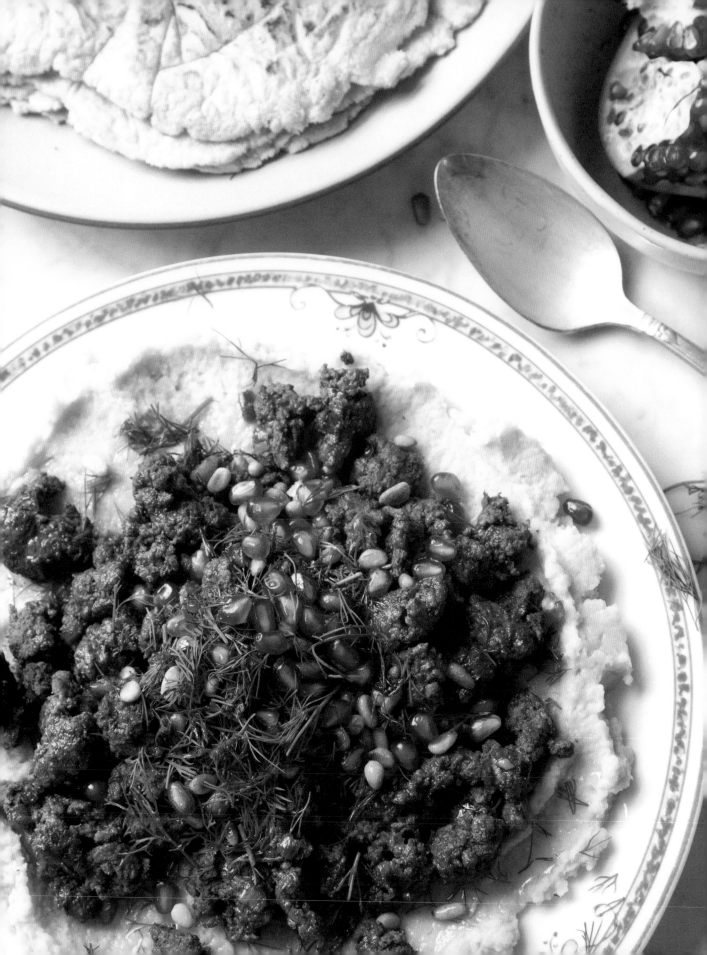

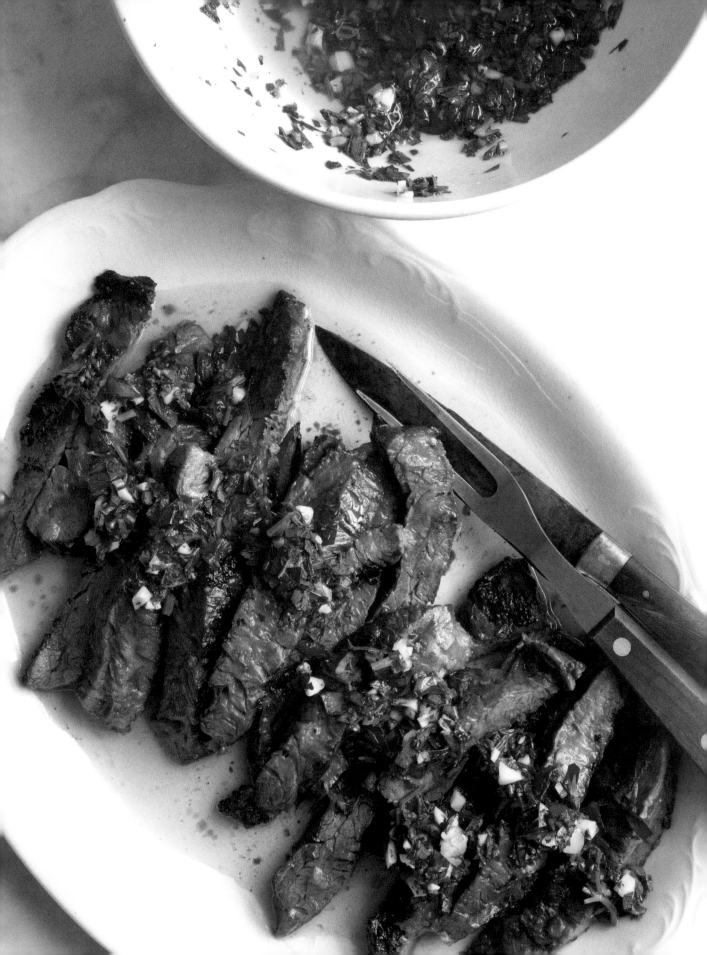

Grilled Skirt Steak with House Chimichurri

Skirt steak is a cut of beef known for its intense beefy flavor rather than for its tenderness. However, there are a few easy steps you can take to ensure moist, succulent steak! Start by dry-brining it in the fridge for 4 hours with salt and a touch of sugar. The salt will tenderize and season the meat, and the sugar will help ensure the meat takes on a nice crust when it gets seared, locking in precious juices. The other important trick to know is that you must slice it *against* the grain. By doing this, you're shortening the muscle strands, making it much easier to chew. It really works. This steak is thin and cooks quickly, so it's perfect for a quick weeknight dinner.

Mix the salt and sugar in a small bowl.

Season the steak on both sides and place in a baking dish in the fridge, uncovered, for 4 hours, flipping once halfway through.

Remove the steak from the fridge and allow to reach room temperature for about an hour. Pat it dry with paper towels.

Depending on the size of your steak, cut it in half or into 3 pieces, each about 4 to 6 inches long.

Heat a cast-iron skillet over medium-high. We want this pan HOT, so it may take as much as 5 minutes. When the pan begins to smoke, carefully add the ghee and oil, let the fat heat up until it ripples in the pan, then add the first piece of steak. Don't touch it. Cook for 2 to 3 minutes, until the underside has a dark crust, then flip it and cook for another minute for medium-rare, or to your liking. Repeat until all the cuts of steak are cooked. Set them aside to rest for 5 to 10 minutes. Slice the steak against the grain into ½-inch-thick strips, then serve with chimichurri.

Serves 4

2 teaspoons kosher sea salt

1 teaspoon coconut sugar (or brown sugar)

1 pound skirt steak

1 tablespoon ghee, plus more if needed

1 tablespoon extra-virgin olive oil

House Chimichurri (page 5)

Swap It
Instead of (or in addition to) the chimichurri, you can serve these steaks with Cherry Tomato Confit (page 18) or Green Onion Salsa (page 6).

Slow-Roasted Ribs with Sticky Plum BBQ Sauce

This dish reminds me of the hoisin spareribs we would order from Chinese takeout when I was a kid growing up in New York City. I like to use baby back ribs instead, because they are more tender than spareribs—and with these, the meat just falls off the bone. The trick here is a low-and-slow roasting method. If you want to make these in advance, you can roast them, let them cool, and refrigerate until you're ready to reheat. Then you can slather them in barbecue sauce, broil, and serve.

Preheat the oven to 275°F, and adjust an oven rack 8 inches below the heating element.

Using a small sharp knife, remove any thin membrane that still might be covering the bony side of the ribs. Place the ribs on a large baking sheet and season both sides generously with salt and pepper. With the meaty side facing up, slather both racks with the mustard.

Cover the pan tightly with foil and bake for 2½ to 3½ hours, or until the meat is falling off the bone. Check the ribs every 15 minutes or so beginning at 2½ hours.

When the ribs are done, remove the foil and brush each rack with the barbecue sauce on the side facing up.

Broil on high, until the sauce begins to caramelize, 4 to 5 minutes, checking every minute or so. Keep an eye on it!

Serve immediately, sprinkled with the green onions and any extra barbecue sauce on the side.

Serves 4 to 6

2 racks baby back pork ribs
(2 to 2½ pounds each)

Kosher sea salt

Freshly ground black pepper

¼ cup country-style
Dijon mustard

⅓ cup Sticky Plum BBQ Sauce
(page 26), or as needed

¼ cup sliced green onions,
for garnish

Tip
If you're allergic to mustard,
you can simply omit it.

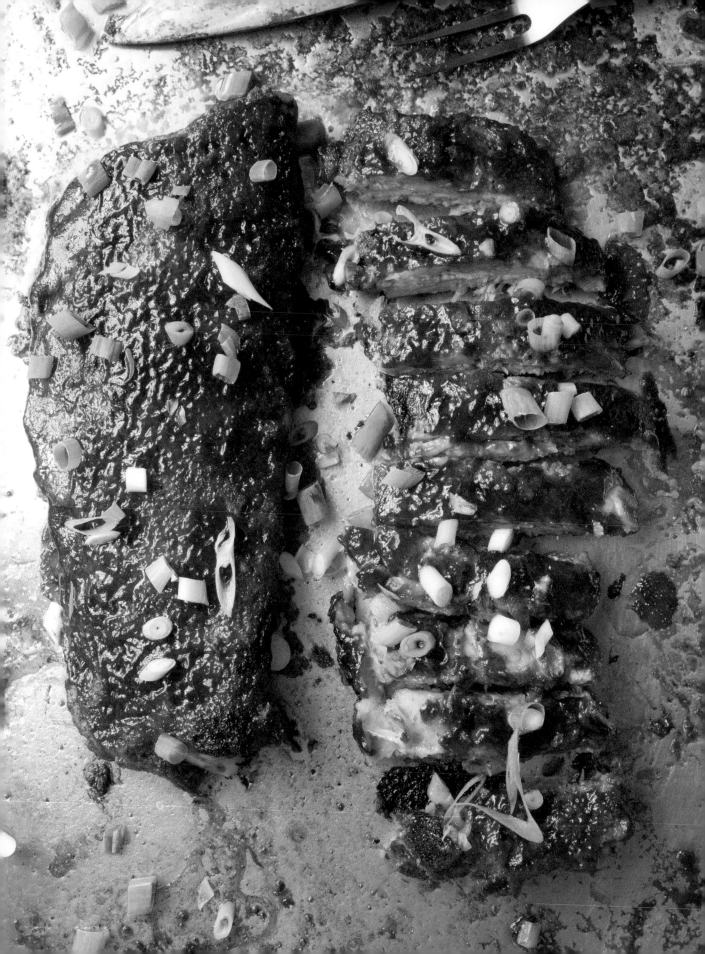

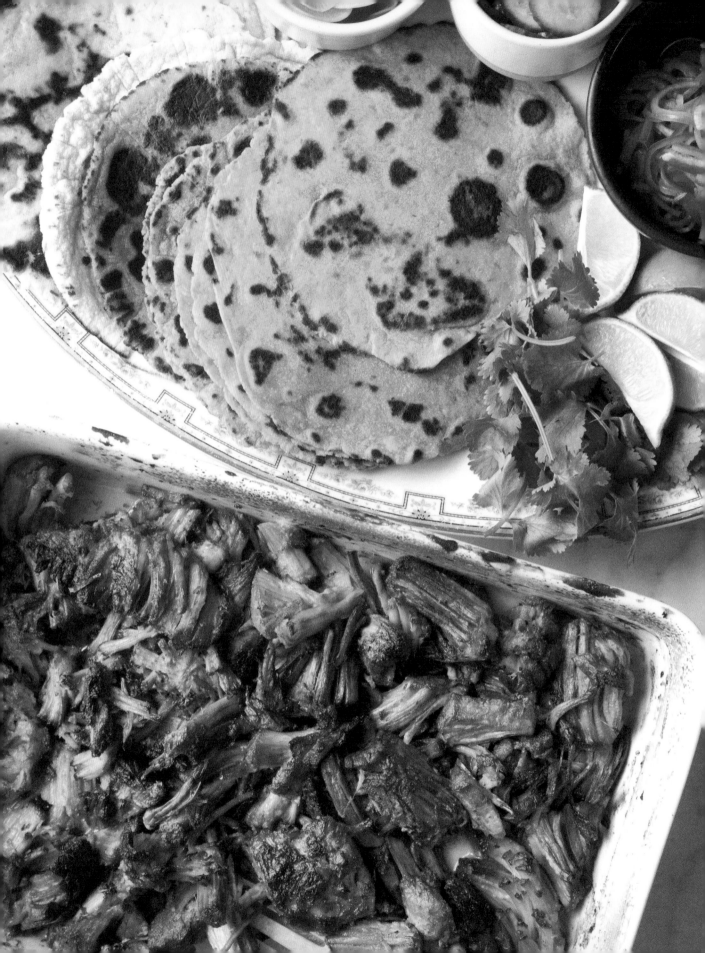

Carnitas

With an initial cooking process similar to that of pork confit, this version of carnitas is cooked low and slow, allowing the meat to tenderize and steep in its own fat, which we help along by adding a little olive oil. And it's not so hard; you just cube the meat and tuck it into a snug baking dish with aromatics, spices, and whole citrus. Perfect for feeding a crowd, the warm spices and rustic presentation make it the ultimate easy-to-make comfort food.

Preheat the oven to 275°F, and set the top rack about 8 inches from the heating element.

Place the pork in a 9-by-13-inch baking dish.

In a small bowl, combine the salt, oregano, cumin, and cloves and mix with 1 tablespoon of the olive oil to form a paste. Rub this mixture over the pork, making sure to coat all the pieces well.

Squeeze the juice from the orange pieces all over the pork, and tuck them into the baking dish along with the onion quarters, garlic cloves, cinnamon stick, and bay leaves. Pour 1/3 cup of the olive oil over everything, cover tightly with aluminum foil, and place in the oven. Cook for 3½ hours, or until the meat is pull-apart tender.

Remove the pork from the oven and let it rest, uncovered, for 10 minutes. Discard the onions, oranges, cinnamon stick, and bay leaves. Transfer the pork to a plate, and strain the remaining cooking juices into a bowl. Place the pork back in the baking dish.

Preheat the oven broiler to high. Use a couple of forks to shred the pork by pulling it apart. Using a large spoon, skim the fat off the top of the juices (or use a fat separator), and drizzle the fat back over the pulled pork. Place the baking dish back in the oven and broil on high for 3 to 5 minutes, or until everything is crispy and dark golden brown. Take the baking dish out, stir the meat, and put it back in the oven again to finish crisping everything up, about another 3 minutes. Spoon some of the leftover juices over the meat to moisten.

Serve the carnitas in tortillas, topped with cilantro and a squeeze of lime.

Serves 4 to 6

3 pounds boneless pork shoulder, cut into 3-inch cubes

1 tablespoon kosher sea salt

2 teaspoons dried oregano

1 teaspoon ground cumin

⅛ teaspoon ground cloves

⅓ cup plus 1 tablespoon extra-virgin olive oil, divided

1 orange, quartered

1 medium yellow onion, peeled and quartered

6 cloves garlic

1 cinnamon stick

2 bay leaves

Tortillas (such as Cassava Tortillas, page 197, or Sweet Potato Tortillas, page 197), chopped cilantro, and lime wedges, for serving

Sauce It
For a full-on taco night, try serving these with Chipotle Aioli (page 21), Smashed Cumin Guacamole (page 22), and Quick Pickled Red Onions (page 28).

Tip
You should have approximately 1 cup of cooking liquid left after cooking these. Save it to make an instant cup of soup! Just reheat it on the stove, adding some fresh spinach and mushrooms to the flavorful broth.

Grass-Fed Rack of Lamb

The first time I ever cooked for my husband, I made rack of lamb. I ate with my hands and chewed on the bones, while he watched with amusement and ate his own lamb using a knife and fork. Eventually he got jealous with how much more I seemed to be enjoying my dinner, so he gave it a go and has never looked back. This is elegant enough to serve at the holidays and simple enough for a weeknight dinner. A rack of lamb elevates any occasion, and you can scale this up or down effortlessly to accommodate any party size. (And if you ask me, it's always okay to eat with your hands.) If you can't find a rack that comes frenched, ask your butcher to do it for you.

In a mini food processor (or chopping by hand), combine the rosemary, garlic, and salt. Pulse a few times, until the garlic and rosemary are broken down. Scrape down the sides of the bowl, add the mustard and olive oil, and process again until a thick paste forms.

Rub the mixture over the fatty side of the lamb racks, and set them on a baking sheet lined with parchment paper, fat side up. Refrigerate overnight, uncovered. (If you're short on time, you can refrigerate for a minimum of 4 hours.)

When you're ready to cook the lamb, remove it from the fridge and allow to reach room temperature, about an hour. Preheat the oven to 450°F.

Roast the lamb for 25 minutes on the center rack, or until a thermometer inserted into the center of the roast measures 125°F for medium-rare.

Remove the lamb from the oven and transfer to a cutting board. Cover loosely with foil and allow to rest for 10 minutes.

Slice between every pair of rib bones to make thick chops, then transfer to a serving dish and serve immediately.

Serves 4 to 6

3 tablespoons chopped fresh rosemary

2 tablespoons chopped garlic (from about 5 cloves)

2 teaspoons kosher sea salt

1 tablespoon country-style Dijon mustard

3 tablespoons extra-virgin olive oil

2 (roughly 1-pound) racks of grass-fed lamb, frenched

Sauce It
Serve with the Cilantro-Mint Chutney (page 7) or Coconut Yogurt Tzatziki (page 31).

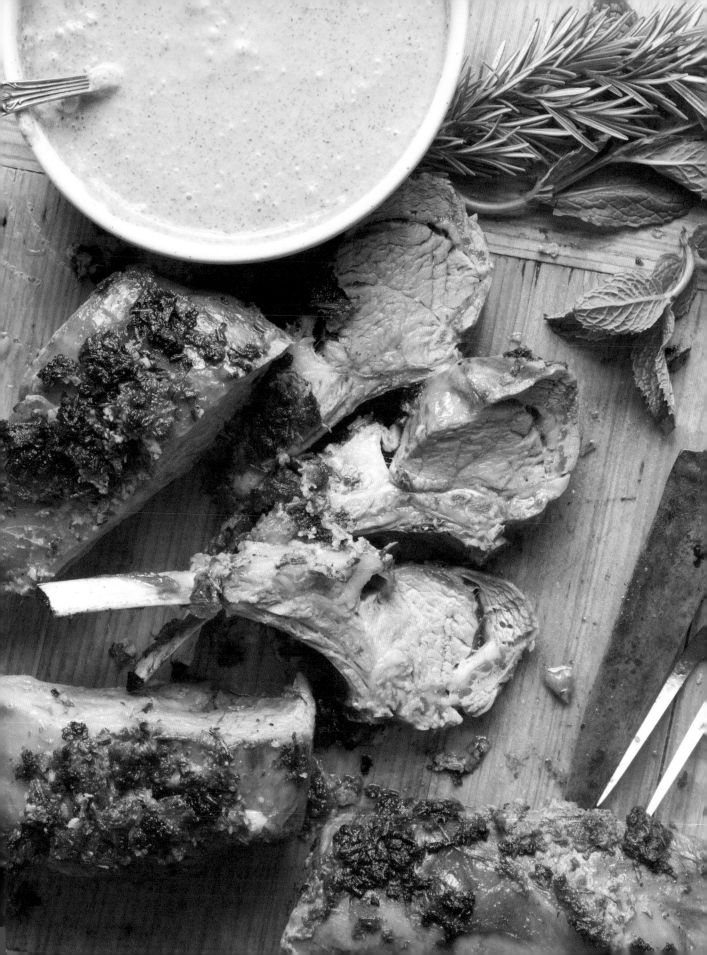

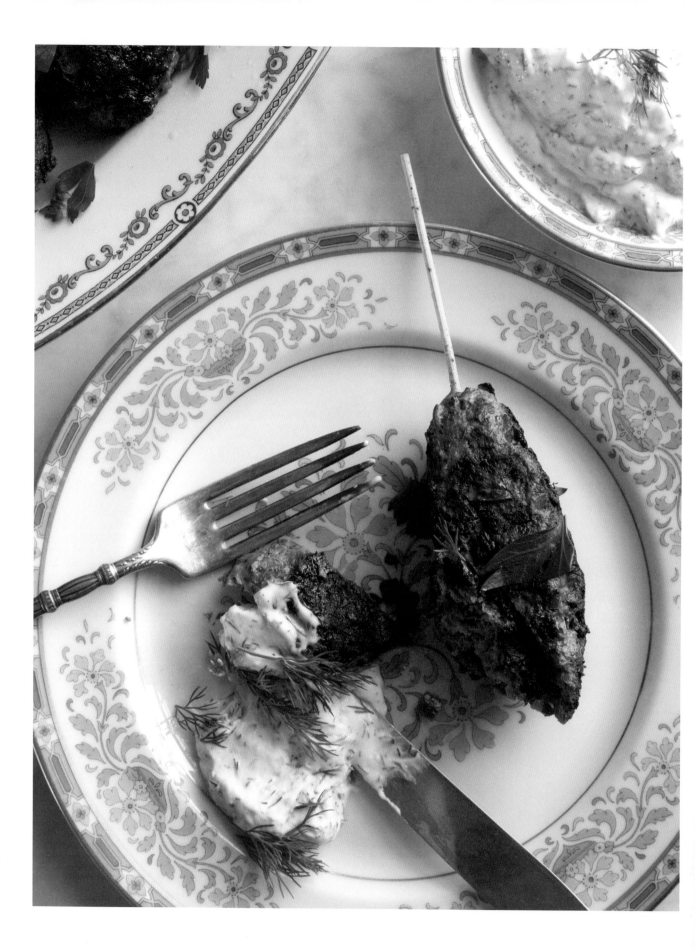

Lamb Koftas

Nearly every major country has its own version of a meatball, with recipes dating as far back as the 11th century. Historically, they started as something very simple, consisting of only ground meat and spices—meaning they were inherently allergen-friendly. *Koftas*, kebabs, and the other meaty skewers of the Middle East tend to be great options for people with food sensitivities because there aren't usually bread crumbs or eggs involved. Generously seasoned with warm, nutty spices and fresh herbs, these meatballs are chock-full of bold flavor and super easy to make—which means even those without dietary concerns are still excited when koftas are on the table. This recipe calls for cooking on a grill pan indoors, but you could also throw these on an outdoor grill as well.

Begin by soaking 8 (6- or 10-inch) wooden skewers in 1 inch of water in a bowl while you prepare the meatball mixture. If you're using metal skewers, skip this step.

In a large bowl, combine the lamb with the onions, garlic, and all the herbs and spices. Mix everything thoroughly by hand. Divide the mixture in half and continue dividing until you have 8 portions that are roughly the same size.

Form each portion into the shape of a sausage about 1½ inches in diameter, then skewer it the long way.

Heat a large square grill pan on medium until hot, about 4 minutes. Add 1 tablespoon of the olive oil and place 4 skewers in the pan, pressing gently and flattening them slightly with tongs. Cook for 5 minutes, until nicely browned, then turn them over and cook for another 5 minutes, until browned on the other side. Turn again to cook on one thin side for 2 minutes, then turn again on the other side to cook for a final 2 minutes. When you're sure that all sides have been seared and browned, transfer the koftas to a serving plate. Repeat with the remaining kebabs.

Let the koftas rest for 10 minutes, then serve with Coconut Yogurt Tzatziki (page 31).

Makes 8 large kebabs

2 pounds ground lamb

½ medium red onion, diced (about 1 cup)

3 large cloves garlic, minced

½ cup finely chopped fresh parsley

¼ cup finely chopped fresh mint

1½ teaspoons kosher sea salt

1 teaspoon ground cumin

1 teaspoon ground cinnamon

2 tablespoons extra-virgin olive oil, divided

Coconut Yogurt Tzatziki (page 31)

Tip
You can also add ½ cup of chopped raisins to the meatball mixture for extra sweetness.

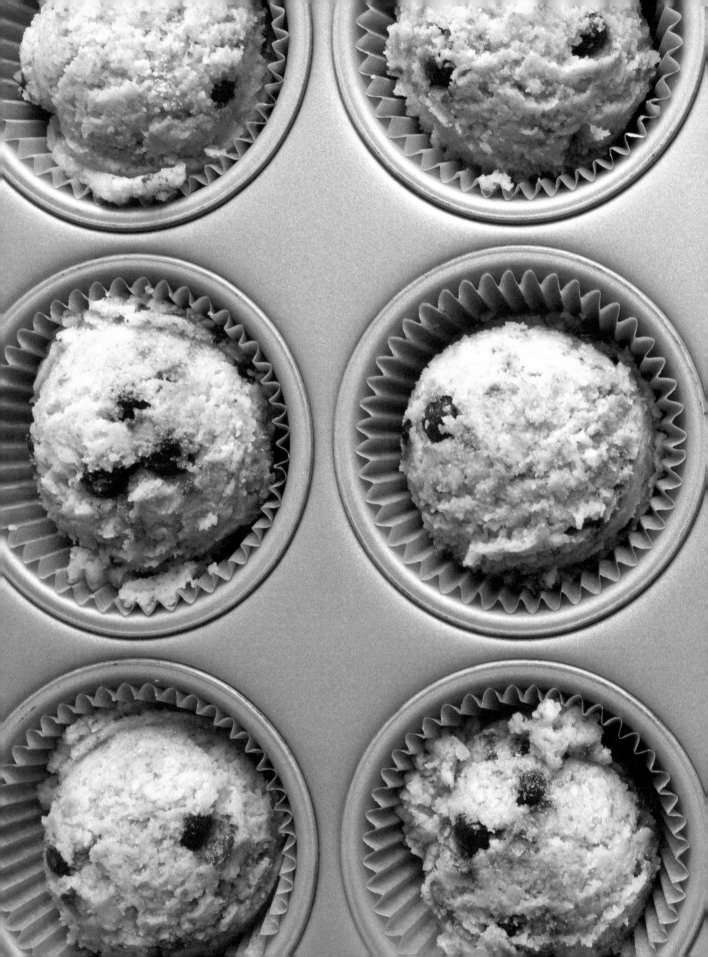

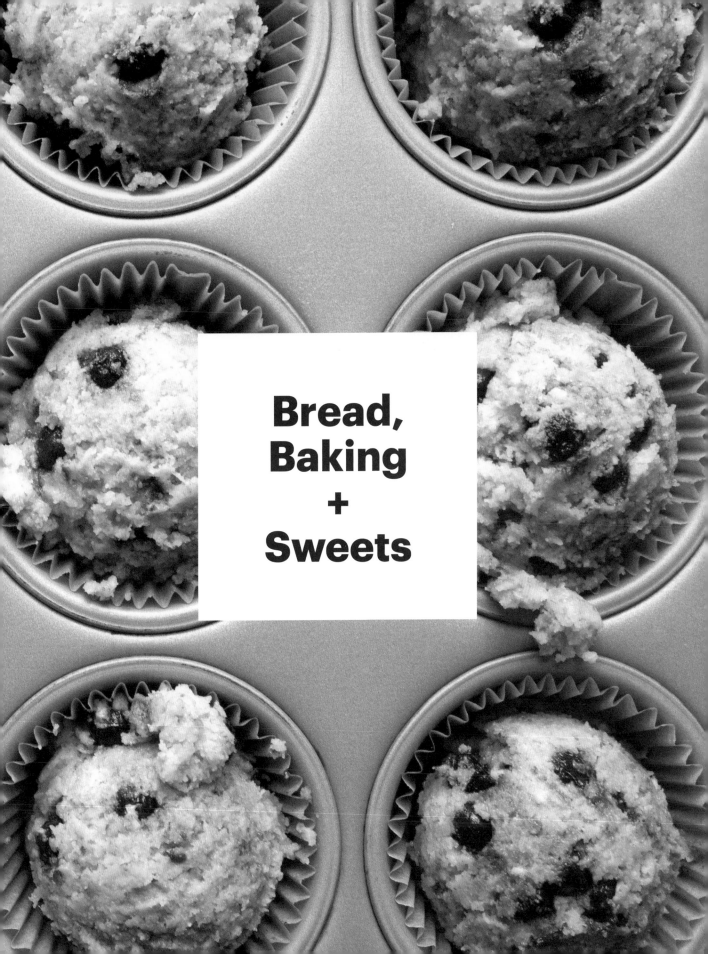

Bread,
Baking
+
Sweets

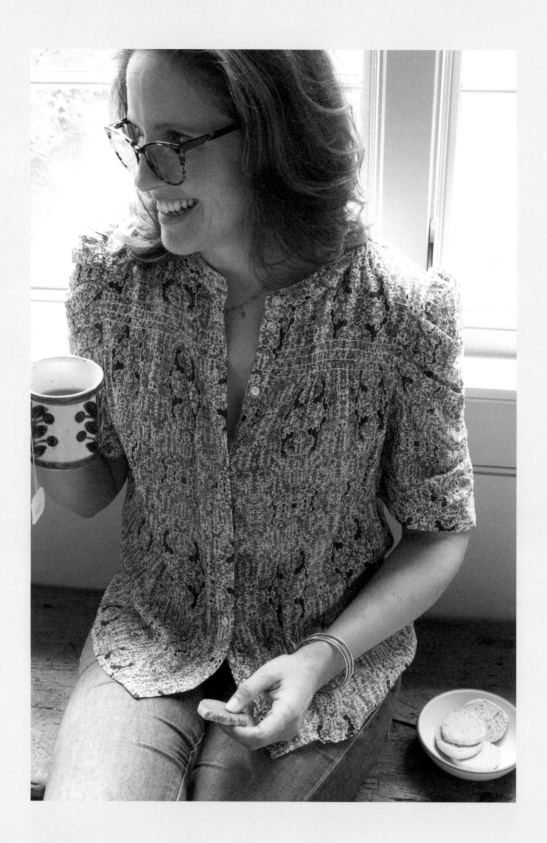

Have Your Cake and Eat It Too

It all started with a bread recipe. In 2018, I decided to publish my blog, *The Kitchen Commune*. It was a place where I could share the various recipes that I had been developing over the decade-plus-long journey of using a food-as-medicine approach to heal my body. This particular loaf of bread was a labor of hormonal love. I took the principles of seed-cycling, which is a holistic method of balancing female hormones by eating specific seeds during the two phases of the menstrual cycle, and applied them to baked goods. (Sexy stuff!) I developed two delicious loaves of bread that used the seeds, which made it easy to incorporate the seed-cycling practice into daily life. Let's just say the ladies loved it!

While the hormonal benefits were great, what I loved most about the breads was simply that they were breads, which I hadn't been eating. Baked goods are probably the most nostalgic and comforting foods we eat. When you're changing your diet for health reasons, they're often the first to go, but we miss them. I've found that for me, it's super important to find delicious and familiar substitutes. I know that I will eat birthday cake, no matter how strict I am, so it might as well be one that's made with ingredients that are nutritious and easier to digest. If you're going to make lasting changes to your health, you need to have some good bread and cake recipes in your back pocket, like the Grain-Free Vegan Boule (page 201) and Grain-Free Dark Chocolate Cake with Chocolate Sweet Potato Frosting (page 215). It doesn't hurt to have a good Shortbread Tea Biscuit (page 220) or Vanilla Ice Cream (page 225) recipe on hand either!

You are human, after all, and it's safe to say that you will need to ultimately find a healthy balance in your food choices so that what you eat can be nutritious but also joyful and sustainable. I've been on the all-or-nothing train. It led me down the self-judgment spiral to nowhere, which didn't serve my health at all! Allowing yourself small indulgences that are made with healthful ingredients is a smarter way to have your cake and eat it too.

Flatbreads

I adapted this recipe from a Milk Street kitchen flatbread recipe to make it grain- and dairy-free. Its sturdy, pliable texture holds up well to all kinds of toppings. You can also tear it apart and use it as a scoop with dip, like you would naan or pita. It's worth mentioning that not all cassava flours are alike, and some can produce a runny mess. You may need to test a few brands before you find the right one; I like Otto's. This dough is also more delicate to handle than traditional naan dough, so we roll it out with parchment paper and use a spatula to flip it instead of tongs. It's easy once you get the hang of it!

Whisk the yogurt, ½ cup of the water, and olive oil together in a measuring cup.

Add the flour, salt, and baking powder to the bowl of a food processor and pulse a few times until well combined. With the processor running, add the yogurt mixture and the remaining ½ cup of water. If needed, add more water 1 tablespoon at a time, and pulse until the dough balls up. If it doesn't ball up, turn it out onto a cutting board lightly dusted with cassava flour and knead it briefly by hand; it will come together.

Divide the dough into 4 equal pieces, and roll each one into a ball. Cover the balls with plastic wrap and let rest for 15 minutes.

Heat a large cast-iron or nonstick skillet over medium-high until it is screaming hot, about 5 minutes. You should see some very light wisps of smoke coming off the pan.

Roll out a ball of dough to a 10-inch round between 2 pieces of parchment paper on your countertop or a large cutting board. Carefully remove the paper: First, peel back the top piece of parchment paper and set it aside for the remaining dough. Lift the remaining dough and paper onto one open palm, with the dough facing up, and flip it into your other hand; then gently peel off the remaining piece of parchment paper. Flip the dough into the pan. Cook undisturbed for 1 to 2 minutes, or until lightly charred. Using a rubber spatula, flip the dough and cook for another minute, or until charred and slightly puffed up. Transfer to a plate and cover with a dish towel. Repeat until all the flatbreads are cooked.

Makes 4 (10-inch) flatbreads

- ½ cup unsweetened, plain Greek-style coconut yogurt (such as Cocojune Pure Coconut)
- 1 cup water, divided, plus 2 more tablespoons if needed
- 2 tablespoons extra-virgin olive oil
- 2 cups cassava flour (such as from Otto's), plus more for dusting
- 1 teaspoon kosher sea salt
- 1½ teaspoons aluminum-free baking powder

Tip
A thick yogurt works better in this recipe. If your yogurt is thin, try straining it in cheesecloth over a bowl to remove excess water.

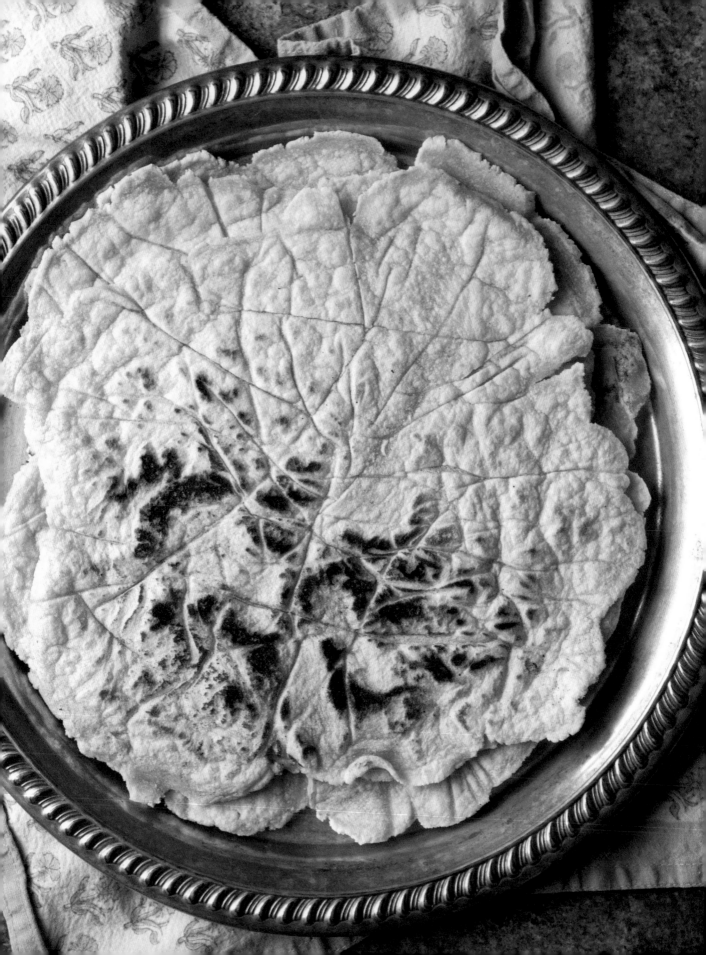

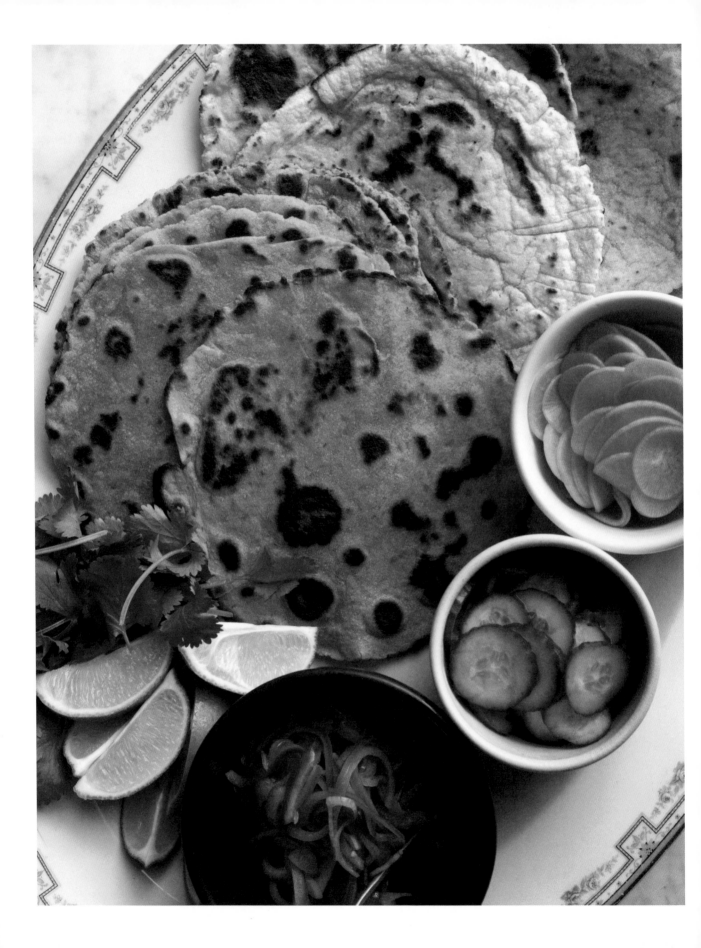

Tortillas

Have you ever made your own tortillas? You can roll these out between two pieces of parchment paper on a cutting board, but I think it's worth making the small investment in a tortilla press. It guarantees even thickness every time, and frankly, it's just more fun. These are a grain-free revelation. The texture is perfectly familiar. Just like a traditional flour tortilla, these are soft and pliable and cook up nice and toasty with charred brown spots. They hold up well, too, keeping your fillings safe and secure. Go ahead and pile it on!

Sweet Potato Tortillas

Preheat the oven to 450°F.

Prick the sweet potatoes all over with a fork and place on a small baking sheet. Roast in the oven for 45 minutes, or until completely tender.

Remove the potatoes from the oven and allow to cool slightly, about 10 minutes. Cut the skin open and scoop out the flesh into a 1-cup measuring cup; set anything extra aside.

In a small bowl, whisk together the cassava flour and salt.

In a medium bowl, add the measured sweet potato and olive oil and mix with a rubber spatula. Add the dry ingredients and fold together until a dough forms. Finish kneading in the bowl by hand until the dough is smooth like Play-Doh, about 30 seconds.

Makes 8 tortillas

1 to 2 sweet potatoes

1 cup cassava flour (such as from Otto's)

½ teaspoon kosher sea salt

⅓ cup plus 1 tablespoon extra-virgin olive oil

Cassava Tortillas

In a medium bowl, whisk the dry ingredients together. In a small bowl, combine the water and oil. Add the wet ingredients to the dry and fold with a spatula until the dough comes together. Finish kneading in the bowl by hand until the dough is smooth like Play-Doh, about 30 seconds.

Recipe continues

Makes 8 tortillas

1½ cups cassava flour (such as from Otto's)

½ teaspoon granulated garlic

¾ teaspoon kosher sea salt

1 cup plus 2 tablespoons water

¼ cup extra-virgin olive oil

Cooking the Tortillas

Turn the dough out onto a cutting board. Shape it into a log and, using a knife, divide it into 8 equal pieces. Roll each piece into a ball, transfer to a plate, and cover with plastic wrap.

Heat a dry cast-iron skillet (or 2, if you'd like to expedite the process) over medium-high heat until very hot, about 5 minutes. Using a tortilla press lined with 2 pieces of plastic wrap, press a ball to about 7 inches in diameter. Or, if using a rolling pin, roll out a ball between 2 pieces of plastic wrap or parchment paper. Carefully remove the plastic wrap: First, peel back the top piece and set it aside for the remaining dough. Lift the remaining dough and plastic onto one open palm, with the dough facing up, and flip it into your other hand; then gently peel off the remaining piece of plastic.

Flip the dough into the pan. Cook undisturbed until nicely charred with dark brown spots and edges, about 2 minutes; then use a spatula to flip. Cook for another minute, then transfer the tortilla to a clean dish towel and wrap it up to keep warm. Repeat until all the tortillas are cooked.

Serve immediately, or allow to cool, stack between squares of parchment paper, and store in an airtight bag or container in the fridge for up to a week. Reheat in a dry nonstick skillet for 1 minute on each side.

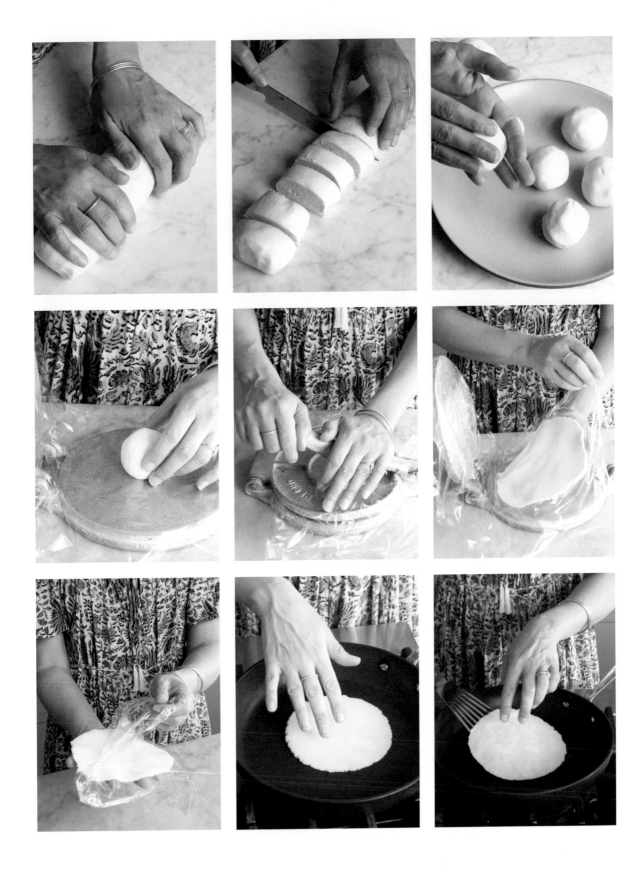

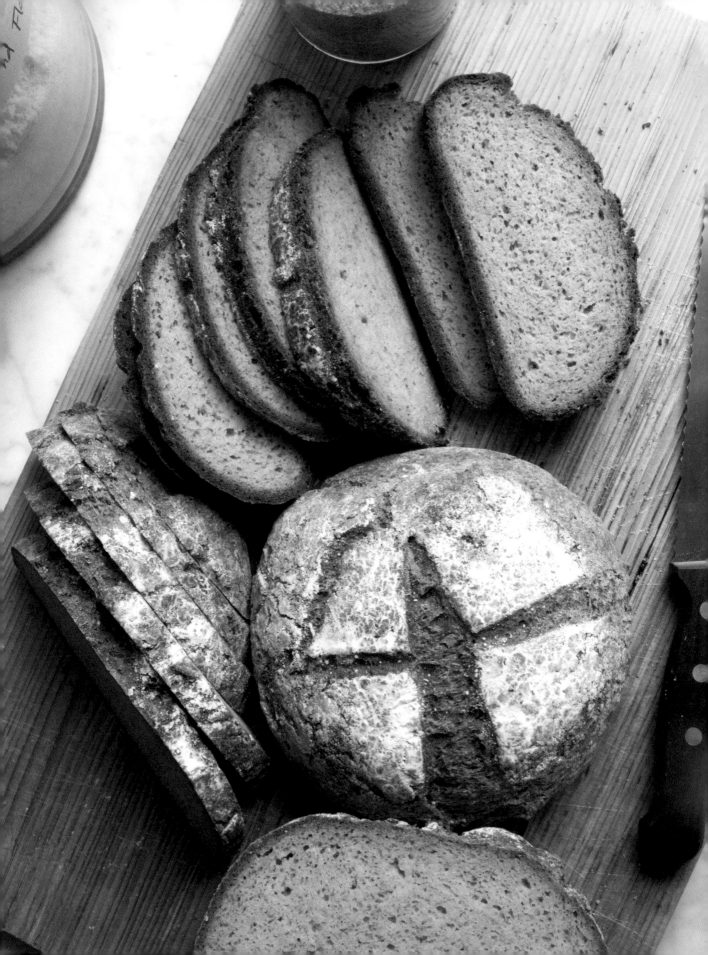

Grain-Free Vegan Boule

I learned so much while developing this precious loaf. I will say that it brought tears to my eyes when I sat down for the first time to enjoy a piece of this hearty, handmade bread. There are no grains, gluten, dairy, eggs, or soy in this recipe. I have journeyed to love the food that loves me back and bread—really, really exciting good bread—was a casualty along the way. Until now!

Here, I am relying solely on oven spring, when the bread first goes into the oven and the loaf expands rapidly before the yeast dies off and the crust sets. We have about the first 20 minutes of baking to get this beauty to rise, and from there, it's just finishing the cooking process. We're skipping over the ever-so-sacred and traditional steps of fermentation and proofing altogether. It sounds quite outrageous, I know, but so is grain-free, vegan bread! It also happens to be less time-consuming and doesn't require a stand mixer. The only extra time here is what happens afterward. You really need to let this bread cool completely. A minimum of 6 hours is good, but overnight is ideal.

While this recipe is quite simple, it is important to follow the directions exactly. I don't usually bake with metric measurements, but I've found that for this bread, weighing out the flour and water in grams helps to ensure success.

Preheat the oven to 350°F. Line a baking sheet with parchment paper and dust it with about a tablespoon of the arrowroot flour.

In a large bowl, combine the almond flour, 1 cup arrowroot flour, and salt, and whisk together very well, making sure all of the ingredients are thoroughly incorporated.

In a 2-cup or larger liquid measuring cup, whisk the water and yeast together, then add the maple syrup and whisk. Add the psyllium husk and vinegar and whisk again. Set this aside to gel for about 3 to 5 minutes, until thickened to the consistency of thick apple sauce, whisking occasionally.

Recipe continues

Makes 1 boule

1 cup (130 grams) arrowroot flour, plus 3 tablespoons more for dusting

2 cups (250 grams) superfine blanched almond flour

1½ teaspoons kosher sea salt

1 cup (240 grams) room-temperature water

2 teaspoons gluten-free active dry yeast (such as Fleischmann's)

2 tablespoons maple syrup

¼ cup (25 grams) whole psyllium husk

1 tablespoon apple cider vinegar

Tip
To make garlic toast, cut thick slices and put in the toaster. Rub toast with a clove of raw garlic, drizzle with extra-virgin olive oil or smear with ghee, and sprinkle with kosher sea salt.

Add the thickened wet mixture to the dry ingredients, making sure to scrape all of it out of the measuring cup with a rubber spatula. Fold the batter together. It will be dry at first, but continue folding, mixing, and scraping down the sides of the bowl with the spatula. It will come together and eventually the dough will ball up. This may take a few minutes, and you might even break a sweat.

Lightly dust a cutting board or work surface with another tablespoon of the arrowroot flour and turn the dough out onto it. Gently flatten the dough into a roughly 8-inch disk and then fold the edges up and over the center of the dough, working with your palms (as opposed to your fingers) to fold about a quarter of the dough into the center at a time and rotating the dough as you go, like wrapping a package. Once you have completed folding in all four sides, flip the dough so it's seam side down and shape into a tight round ball by tucking any unrounded sections underneath.

Transfer the dough ball to the floured parchment paper. Dust the top of the loaf with the remaining arrowroot flour and score a 2-inch X, about ¼-inch deep, onto the center of the top of the loaf, using a small sharp knife. This will allow for even expansion and help prevent tears.

Bake the bread for 60 minutes at 350°F, then lower the oven temperature to 325°F and bake for 20 minutes. The bread will be golden brown and will sound hollow when you (carefully!) thump the bottom.

Remove the bread from the oven and let it cool for 30 minutes, then transfer to a wire rack to cool completely for a minimum of 6 hours (or, preferably, overnight), covered with a dish towel.

Store at room temperature wrapped tightly in parchment paper. You can also slice the entire loaf and freeze it in a large ziplock bag with small pieces of parchment between the slices, and just toast it from frozen as needed.

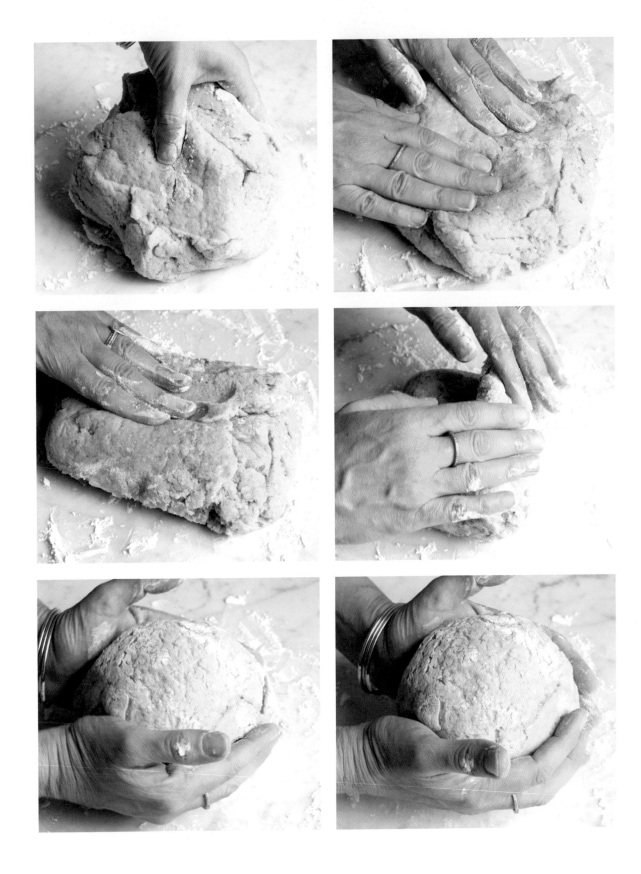

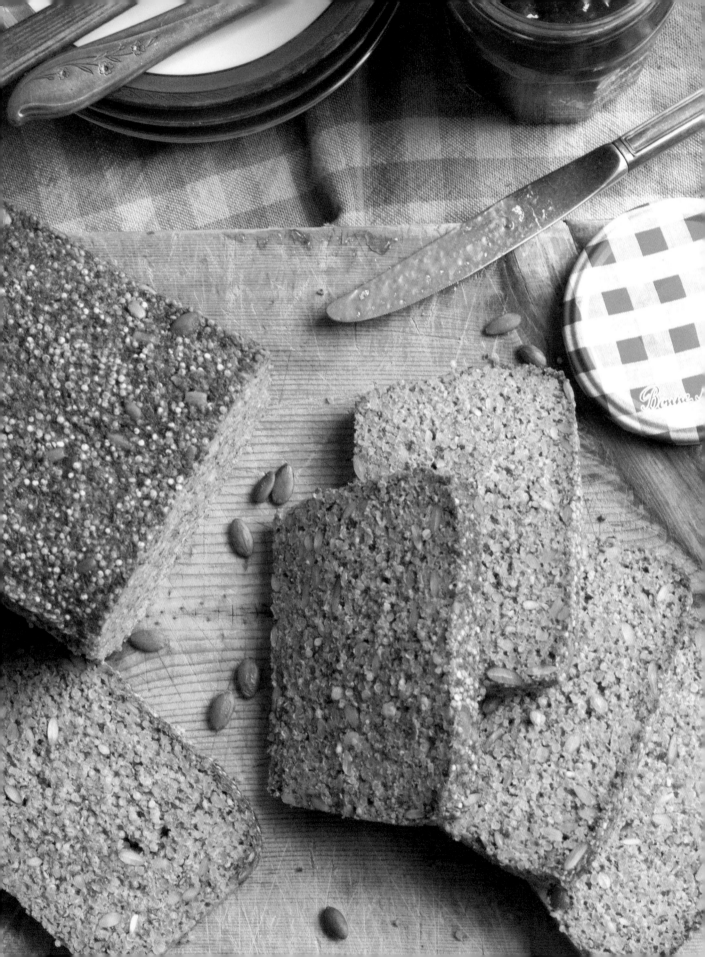

Nut + Seed Bread

This was the first recipe that I published on my blog, *The Kitchen Commune*. I developed this bread with hormone balance in mind. It's chock-full of fiber and extremely nutrient-dense. It's best served thick-cut and open-faced, like a tartine. Toasted or not, it's filling and delicious with all different kinds of toppings, both savory and sweet or simply smeared with ghee, honey, and sea salt. From start to finish, this is a 24-hour process, though much of that time is hands-off. I recommend starting in the morning.

Begin by soaking the quinoa for 8 to 12 hours. Drain and rinse the quinoa in a fine-mesh sieve.

Grease an 8-by-4-inch loaf pan with a generous amount of the olive oil.

In a small mixing bowl, whisk together the 2 cups of water, ¼ cup of olive oil, maple syrup, vinegar, and chia seeds.

In a large bowl, whisk together the almond flour, flaxseed, psyllium husks, and salt. Add the drained quinoa and pumpkin seeds. Use a rubber spatula to mix until well combined. Add the remaining wet ingredients and continue folding until completely incorporated. The mixture should be thick and wet.

Scoop the dough into the prepared loaf pan, and gently push it into an even layer with your fingers or the spatula. Sprinkle a few extra pumpkin seeds over the loaf for garnish.

Loosely cover with a cloth napkin or dish towel and let sit overnight on your countertop for 8 to 12 hours.

When you're ready to bake, preheat the oven to 350°F.

Place the loaf pan on the center rack and bake for 1 hour; the bread should be firm to the touch in the center. Cool completely in the loaf pan. To remove, run a dinner knife gently around the edges of the pan and carefully invert the bread onto a cutting board.

To store, wrap in a piece of parchment paper and keep in an airtight bag in the fridge.

Makes 1 (8-by-4-inch) loaf

1¼ cups quinoa

2 cups water

¼ cup extra-virgin olive oil, plus more for greasing

2 tablespoons maple syrup

1 tablespoon apple cider vinegar

2 tablespoons chia seeds

¾ cup blanched almond flour

¾ cup ground flaxseed or flaxseed meal

⅓ cup whole psyllium husks

1 teaspoon sea salt

¾ cup raw pumpkin seeds, plus more for garnish

Tips
Remember, this is a tartine-style bread and works best open-faced. Thicker slices hold up better in the toaster.

This bread freezes beautifully. Wrap in parchment paper, place in an airtight bag, and freeze. To defrost, keep it wrapped and put in the fridge overnight. It should be thawed and ready to go within 24 hours.

Swap It
Substitute sunflower seeds for the pumpkin seeds, or use a combination of both.

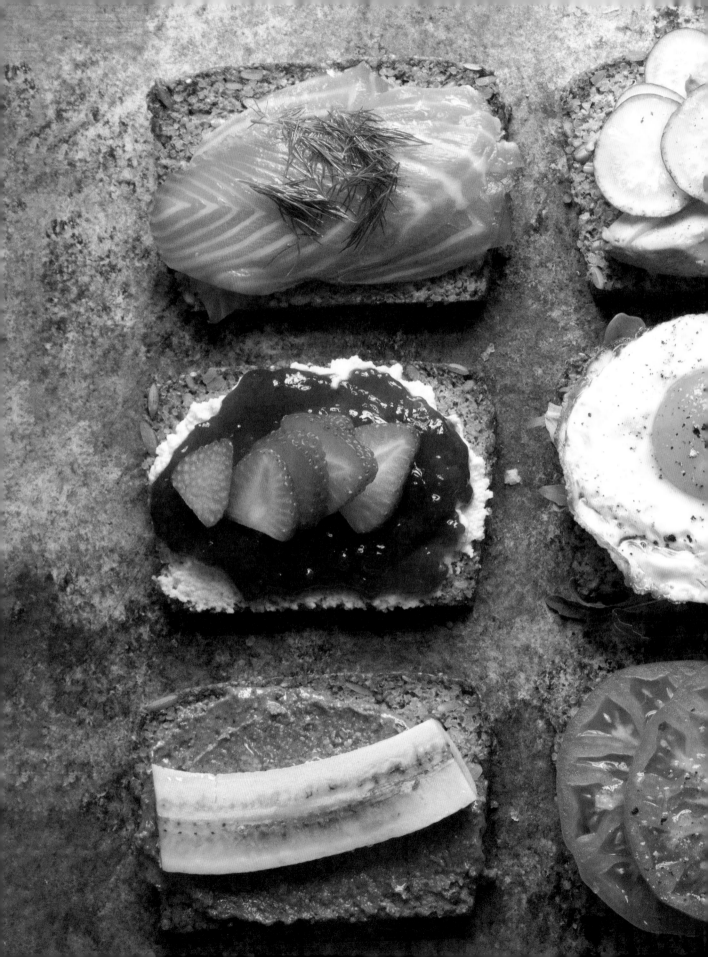

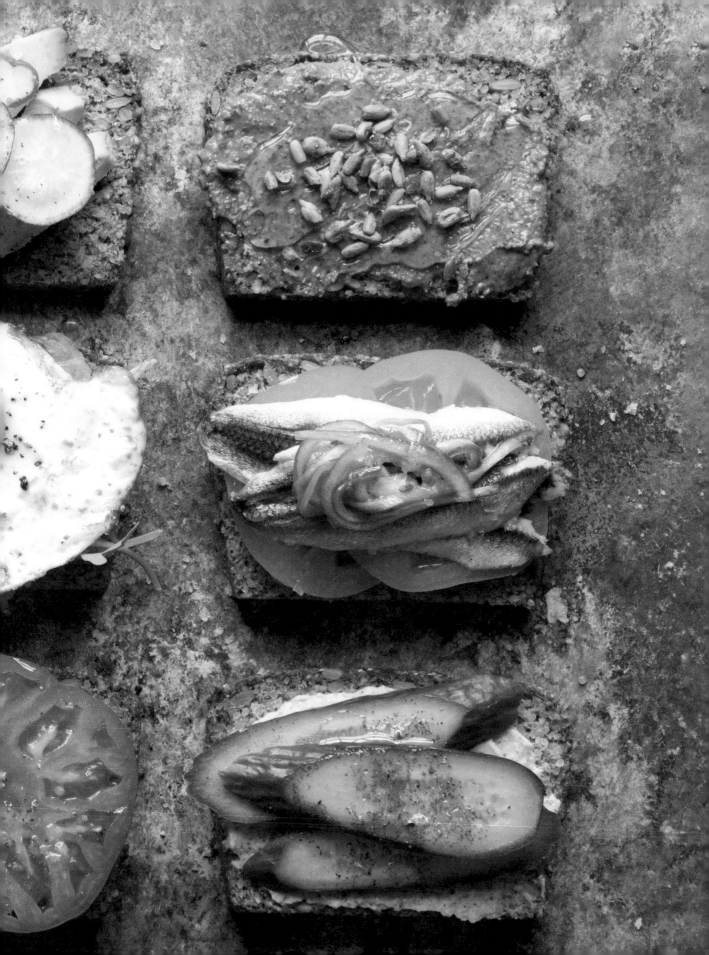

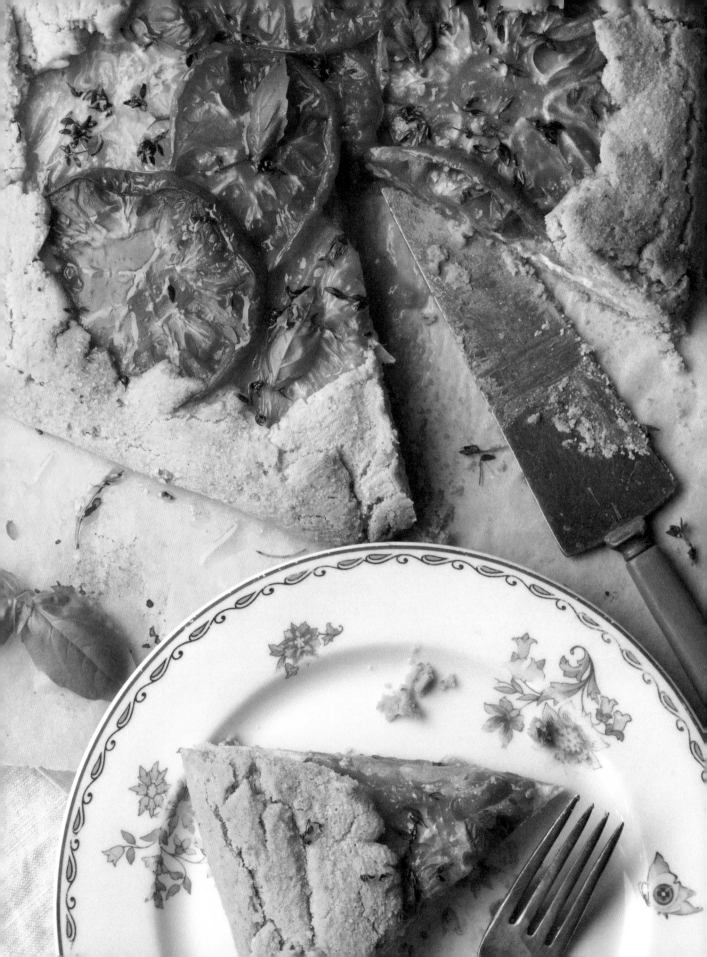

Heirloom Tomato Galette

If you wait until your tomatoes are in season and at their most ripe-and-juicy state before making this galette, you'll thank me—or thank Mother Nature, who will do most of the work for you. This is a great stand-in for pizza if you get the craving! The crust is infused with cheesy nutritional yeast and herbs for added flavor. I love this in the summertime, served with sliced steak or salad for an easy warm-weather dinner alfresco.

Preheat the oven to 375°F, and adjust the oven rack to the center.

Lay your tomato slices out on a plate, season with salt, and allow to develop flavor.

To make the dough: In a large mixing bowl, whisk together all the dry ingredients. In a small cup, mix the wet ingredients, then add them to the dry. Using a rubber spatula, fold and mix thoroughly until the dough comes together and forms a ball. It may take a little time.

Turn the dough out onto a cutting board lined with parchment paper, form into a 6-inch disk, and place a second sheet of parchment paper over the dough. Roll it out until it's about 12 inches in diameter and ¼ inch thick. Don't worry about the shape too much; you should end up with a jagged circle.

Transfer the parchment paper with the dough to a baking sheet and remove the top layer of paper.

Spread the ricotta cheese with a small spatula evenly over the base of the dough like you would pizza sauce, leaving a 1½-inch border. Lay the tomatoes over the cheese, slightly overlapping them, making sure to cover all the cheese. Season the tomatoes with pepper and sprinkle with the fresh thyme.

Recipe continues

Serves 4 to 6

For the Filling

1½ pounds heirloom tomatoes (3 to 4 medium tomatoes), cut into ¼-inch-thick slices

Kosher sea salt

⅔ cup Fresh Almond Ricotta Cheese (page 15)

Freshly ground black pepper

2 teaspoons fresh thyme leaves

2 tablespoons extra-virgin olive oil, divided, plus more for serving

Handful of fresh basil, torn

For the Dough

1½ cups superfine blanched almond flour

⅔ cup arrowroot flour

¼ cup nutritional yeast

1 tablespoon psyllium husk powder

1 teaspoon dried thyme

¼ teaspoon kosher sea salt

¼ cup plus 2 tablespoons water

¼ cup extra-virgin olive oil

To form the galette: This dough is more fragile than traditional dough, so use the parchment paper instead of your hands to form the galette. First, gently lift a roughly 3-inch section of the edge of the dough up and over the tomatoes, folding it so it overlaps the tomatoes by about an inch. Peel the paper back if necessary. Make your way around the whole galette, pleating the dough in successive folds until you have completed the circle and the dough is folded over the entire outer rim of the tomatoes. Press any sections of overlapping dough together firmly as you go. Drizzle 1 tablespoon of olive oil over the tomatoes, and brush the crust with the remaining tablespoon of olive oil.

Bake for 30 minutes, until light golden brown, then broil on high for 2 to 3 minutes to get extra browning on the crust.

Remove from the oven and allow to cool completely, about an hour. Drizzle with olive oil and serve at room temperature, garnished with the basil.

Tips

Drizzle ¼ cup of the House Pesto (page 10) over the ricotta cheese for added flavor, or add a few anchovy fillets.

Cover any leftover galette with plastic wrap and refrigerate for 3 days. Before serving, pop it back in the oven at 350°F for 10 minutes, until warm.

Caramel Pear Galette

I've always been the girl who hunts down caramel apples at the state fair or on the boardwalk, but recently I've come to realize that caramel and pears make an even lovelier combination. This recipe marries my new favorite combo with one of my favorite fuss-free desserts—the galette. I love pie when I'm in need of a good baking meditation, but I adore a galette because you get the same delicious results with a much more laid-back approach. It's pie, but without all the rigmarole. It's a pizza, but made with fruit. You just roll out the dough, dump a pile of luscious fruit smothered in caramel sauce on it, fold up the edges, and bake. It's rustic. You don't have to have super dessert-making skills, but everyone will think you do!

To make the caramel sauce: Combine all the ingredients in a small, heavy-bottomed saucepan and simmer over medium-low heat. Lower the heat to the lowest setting and cook for 10 to 12 minutes until the sauce has reduced by almost half. It should be a little foamy while it cooks. You may have to slide the pot slightly off the burner to get the heat low enough to prevent too much foam.

Remove from the heat, transfer to a small bowl, and allow to cool and thicken, about 20 minutes, stirring occasionally.

Preheat the oven to 375°F.

To make the dough: In a large mixing bowl, whisk together the almond flour, 2/3 cup of the arrowroot flour, psyllium husk powder, and salt. In a small cup, mix all the wet ingredients, then add them to the dry. Using a rubber spatula, fold and mix thoroughly until the dough comes together and forms a ball. It may take a little time, and you may need to scrape off your spatula to incorporate everything. Turn the dough out onto a cutting board lined with parchment paper, then form it into a 6-inch disk.

To make the filling: In a medium bowl, use a rubber spatula to gently toss together the pears and the lemon juice. Add all the caramel sauce except for 2 tablespoons, and the vanilla extract, and gently fold everything together. Sprinkle the remaining 2 tablespoons of arrowroot flour over the filling and gently fold again, making sure to mix thoroughly.

Recipe continues

Serves 8

For the Caramel Sauce

½ cup maple syrup

¼ cup Fresh Almond Cream (page 16)

1 tablespoon ghee

Pinch of kosher sea salt

For the Dough

1¾ cups superfine blanched almond flour

⅔ cup plus 2 tablespoons arrowroot flour, divided

1 tablespoon psyllium husk powder

Pinch of kosher sea salt

3 tablespoons ghee, melted

3 tablespoons maple syrup

2 tablespoons plus 1 teaspoon water

For the Filling

1½ pounds ripe Anjou pears (about 4 pears), skin on, cut into ¼-inch-thick slices

1 teaspoon freshly squeezed lemon juice

1 tablespoon alcohol-free vanilla extract

1 teaspoon coconut sugar

Swap It

For the caramel sauce, you can substitute coconut cream or any heavy cream of your choice for the Fresh Almond Cream.

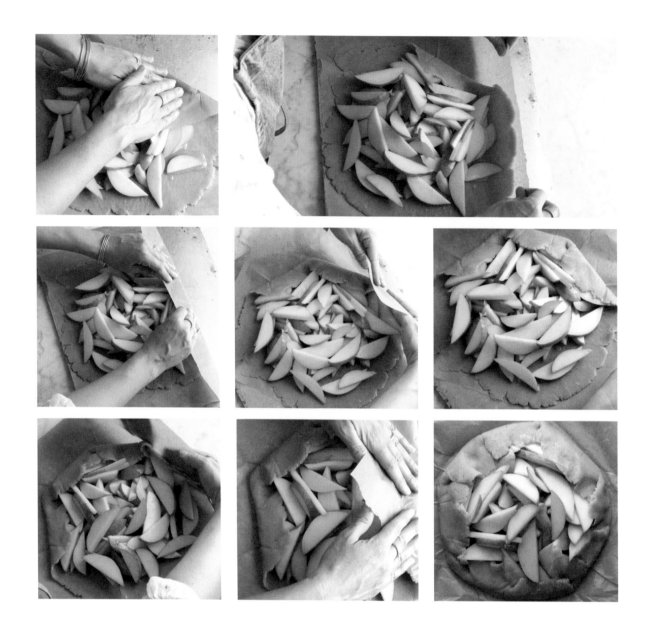

Place a second sheet of parchment paper over the dough, and roll it out until it's about 12 inches in diameter and ¼ inch thick. Don't worry about the shape too much; you should end up with a jagged circle.

Transfer the parchment paper with the dough to a baking sheet, and remove the top layer of paper.

Gently empty the fruit filling from the bowl onto the center of the dough. Spread it out a little, making sure to leave a border of about 1½ inches.

To form the galette: This dough is more fragile than traditional dough, so use the parchment paper instead of your hands to form the galette. First, gently lift a roughly 3-inch section of the edge of the dough up and over the pears, folding it so it overlaps the fruit by about an inch. Peel the paper back if necessary. Make your way around the whole galette, pleating the dough in successive folds until you have completed the circle and the dough is folded over the entire outer rim of the pears. Press any sections of overlapping dough together firmly as you go. Brush the crust with the remaining caramel sauce and sprinkle the coconut sugar over the filling.

Bake for 25 minutes, until the crust is golden brown.

Remove from the oven and allow to cool for 30 minutes before transferring to a serving dish.

To store any uneaten galette, allow to cool completely, cover with plastic wrap, and refrigerate for up to 3 days. Before serving, pop it back in the oven at 350°F for 10 minutes, until warm.

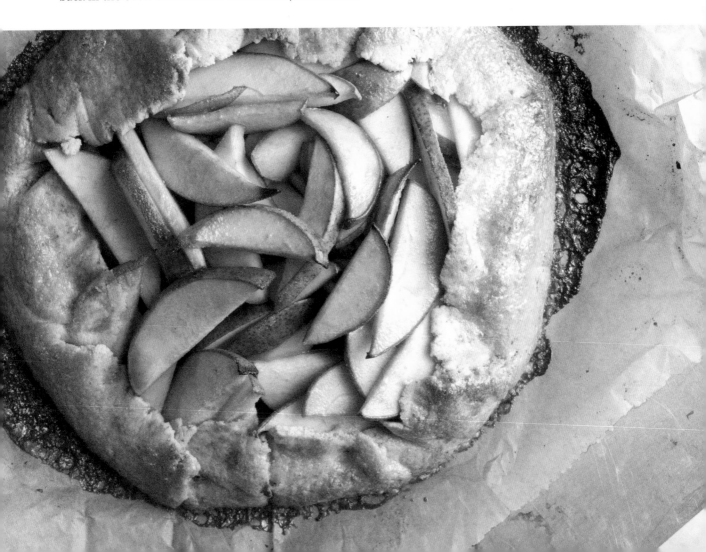

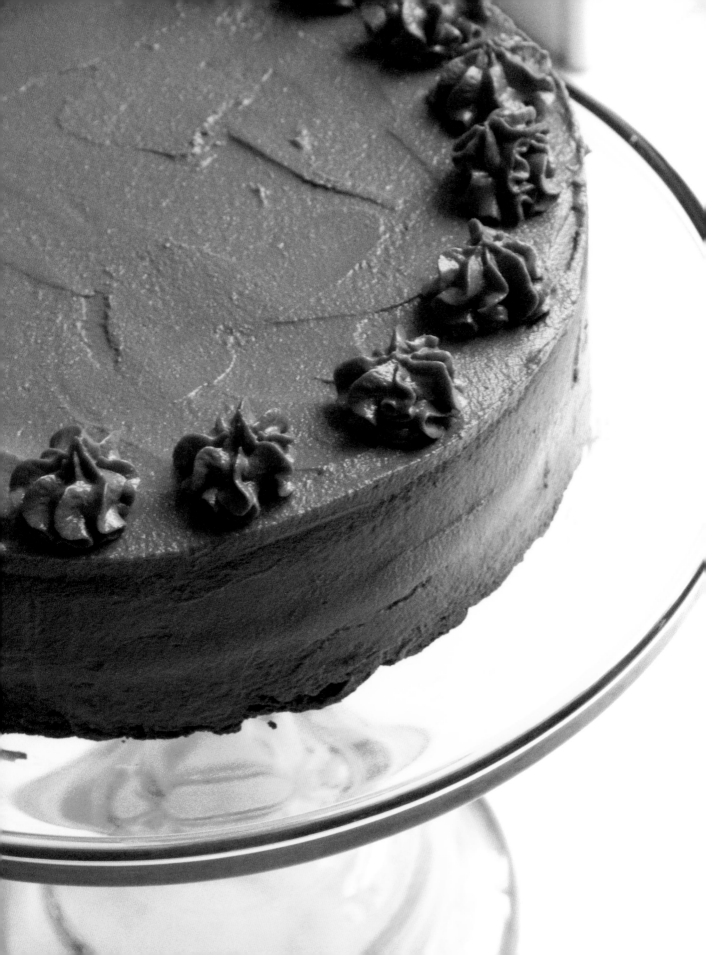

Grain-Free Dark Chocolate Cake with Chocolate Sweet Potato Frosting

The teenagers in my house and the surrounding area have approved this allergen-friendly chocolate cake, right down to its sweet, creamy frosting. The first time I made it, I didn't tell them the frosting was made from vegetables. During the big reveal—after they'd devoured every last bite off the cake platter the way only a group of teens can do—my daughter, who generally hates sweet potatoes, was shocked to learn that the frosting was full of them. We had a good laugh. Sometimes you have to be stealthy when you're introducing new food concepts to people who don't have any allergies. Tell them what's in it after they lick the plate.

In contrast to most cakes, I like this one best chilled.

Preheat the oven to 450°F. Make the frosting first.

Prick the sweet potatoes all over with a fork and place them on a small baking sheet lined with parchment paper. Roast for about 60 minutes, or until completely tender in the center.

Remove the sweet potatoes from the oven and set aside until cool enough to handle, about 10 minutes. Cut the skins open and scoop out the flesh. Measure 2 packed cups of flesh and transfer to the bowl of a food processor. Add the rest of the frosting ingredients and process for about 30 seconds, until a thick-and-creamy frosting forms. Scrape down the sides of the bowl and process again for another 10 seconds, or until smooth. Transfer to an airtight container to cool completely, then cover and place in the fridge for a minimum of 4 hours (or overnight) to set.

To make the cake, preheat the oven to 350°F. Grease 2 (8-inch) cake pans with avocado oil, and line the bottom of each with parchment paper.

Recipe continues

Serves 8

For the Chocolate Sweet Potato Frosting

2 large orange-fleshed sweet potatoes (such as Jewel or Garnet, about 2 pounds total)

½ cup cacao powder

¾ cup maple syrup

¼ cup melted coconut oil

1 tablespoon alcohol-free vanilla extract

Pinch of kosher sea salt

For the Cake

½ cup avocado oil, plus more for greasing the pan

¼ cup ground flaxseed or flaxseed meal

⅔ cup hot water

1 cup superfine blanched almond flour

½ cup cassava flour (such as Otto's)

½ cup coconut flour

2 tablespoons tapioca flour

⅔ cup cacao powder

2 teaspoons aluminum-free baking powder

1 teaspoon baking soda

½ teaspoon kosher sea salt

1 cup almond milk

1 cup maple syrup

1 tablespoon alcohol-free vanilla extract

In a medium bowl, whisk together the flaxseed and hot water and allow to thicken for about 15 minutes, stirring occasionally.

In a large bowl, combine and whisk together all the dry ingredients.

Add the remaining wet ingredients to the flaxseed mixture and whisk together well. Add the wet ingredients to the dry; using a spatula, mix everything well until a thick, smooth batter forms.

Divide the batter evenly between the 2 pans, using the back of a spoon to smooth out the surface of the batter. Bake on the center rack for 30 to 35 minutes, or until a toothpick inserted in the center comes out clean. Let the cakes cool in the pan for 30 minutes, then run a kitchen knife around the edges of each cake to loosen. Invert each cake onto a rack and peel off the parchment paper. Allow to cool completely, about 2 hours. If working ahead, wrap each cake layer individually and tightly in plastic wrap and store at room temperature until you are ready to assemble the cake.

To assemble the cake, transfer the first layer to a cake stand or a serving dish. Add half the chocolate frosting and spread it evenly over the cake with the back of a large spoon. Place the second cake layer on top of the frosted first layer, and add the remaining frosting.

Serve the cake immediately or refrigerate until chilled, about 4 hours, before serving. Store any leftover cake in the fridge for up to 3 days, covered with plastic wrap, making sure to gently press the wrap against the surface of the cake to create an airtight seal.

Carrot Birthday Cake with Cultured Buttercream + Rainbow Sprinkles

A list of some of my favorite things: roast chicken, fried chicken, cheeseburgers, dark chocolate, hot baths, mascara, my bed, Christmas music, Cadbury Creme Eggs, candy corn, peanut butter cups, the Beatles, black tea with milk, Marmite toast, salt, vanilla ice cream with rainbow sprinkles, seat heaters, the sun, the moon, the stars, the ocean, and carrot cake.

Do I eat all the foods on my list? No, not anymore. But I still have very fond memories of them, and I love re-creating as much as I can. Carrot cake is my birthday cake of choice, hands down. I worked hard to get this buttercream just right. The texture is SO spot-on. It's rich and creamy, yet sturdy enough to hold up between the layers. The cold yogurt adds the tang I'm looking for when I think of cream cheese frosting and puts the coconut butter at just the right temperature to firm up an otherwise-thin icing. With less sugar and super nutrient-dense ingredients, this is a cake you can eat with abandon. The buttercream is best at room temperature. This cake can safely sit unrefrigerated for 2 days.

Lastly, I've made the lemon juice in the buttercream optional. I like the subtle flavor of the yogurt as is, but if you'd like to accentuate that, lemon juice works beautifully.

Preheat the oven to 350°F.

Grease 2 (8-inch) nonstick round cake pans with avocado oil, and line the bottom of each with parchment paper.

In a small bowl, whisk together the ground flaxseed and water and allow to thicken for 15 minutes.

In a medium bowl, whisk together the remaining wet ingredients.

In a large bowl, whisk together all the dry ingredients.

Recipe continues

Serves 8

For the Cake

½ cup avocado oil, plus more for greasing the pan

¼ cup ground flaxseed or flaxseed meal

⅔ cup hot water

1 cup full-fat coconut milk

½ cup maple syrup

1 tablespoon alcohol-free vanilla extract

1 tablespoon freshly squeezed lemon juice

1 cup cassava flour (such as Otto's)

½ cup coconut flour

½ cup superfine blanched almond flour

¼ cup coconut sugar

2 teaspoons aluminum-free baking powder

1 teaspoon baking soda

1 teaspoon kosher sea salt

1 tablespoon ground cinnamon

½ teaspoon ground ginger

⅛ teaspoon ground cloves

2 cups grated carrot (from about 3 medium carrots)

½ cup chopped walnuts (optional)

⅓ cup rainbow sprinkles

Add the flaxseed mixture to the wet ingredients and whisk to combine. Add all the wet ingredients to the dry ingredients, using a rubber spatula to mix well. Add the carrots and walnuts (if using) and fold them into the batter. The batter will be thick.

Divide the batter equally between the 2 cake pans, and use a fork to gently spread the batter out into an even layer.

Bake for 30 minutes, or until fragrant and a toothpick inserted in the center comes out clean.

Remove the cakes from the oven and allow to cool completely in the pans, about 2 hours.

To make the buttercream, melt the coconut butter in a small pot over low heat until just soft and creamy, about 2 minutes. Alternatively, you can heat it up in a small bowl in the microwave for 15 to 30 seconds. Transfer the softened coconut butter to the bowl of a stand mixer.

Add all the other ingredients to the bowl and mix on medium-high for about 30 seconds, scraping the sides as necessary. The buttercream should whip up thick and creamy and be spreadable.

To assemble the cake, run a kitchen knife around the edges of each cake to loosen. Invert each cake pan onto a large plate, remove the pan, and peel off the parchment paper if necessary. Transfer the first layer to a cake stand or a serving dish. Add half the buttercream and spread evenly over the cake. Repeat the process with the second layer of cake; place on top of the frosted first layer and add the remaining buttercream. Spread the frosting evenly over the top layer using an icing spatula or the straight back edge of a dinner knife. Decorate with the rainbow sprinkles on top.

Serve the cake immediately, then store at room temperature, covered, up to 2 days.

For the Cultured Buttercream

1 cup raw coconut butter

1 cup coconut oil

1 cup unsweetened, plain Greek-style coconut yogurt (cold; such as Cocojune Pure Coconut)

½ cup maple syrup

2 tablespoons alcohol-free vanilla extract

2 teaspoons fresh lemon juice (optional)

Tip

The buttercream can be made 2 days in advance and stored at room temperature for best results—just whip it again before applying it to the cake.

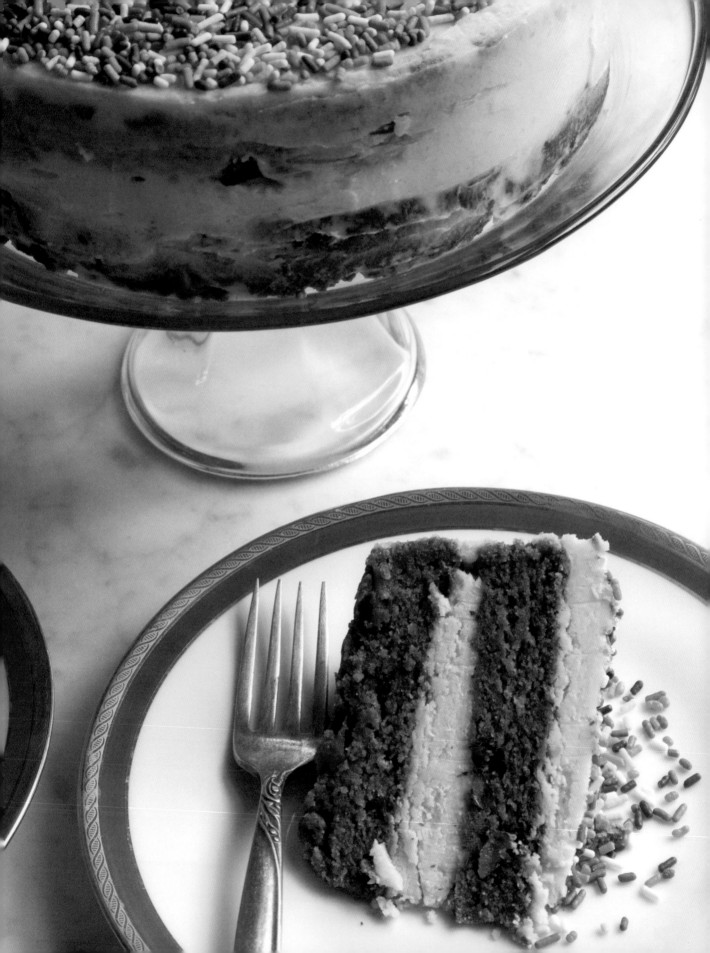

Shortbread Tea Biscuits

Sometimes you just have to have the perfect buttery cookie to dip into your tea or snack on. This one has the flavor and texture of a classic shortbread biscuit, but with much less sugar. I also used ghee instead of butter for two reasons: First, I don't do dairy, but ghee works for me (see Ghee on page xiv). Second, ghee is similar to clarified butter, but made by an extended cooking process, whereby the milk solids in the butterfat are caramelized before being removed, leaving a rich, nutty flavor profile—perfect for shortbread. If you really want to gild the lily, spread these biscuits with your favorite jam or melted chocolate and make cookie sandwiches.

In a small bowl, whisk together the flaxseed meal and the water and allow to thicken.

On a plate large enough to hold 8 separate tablespoons of ghee, measure the ghee, placing each tablespoon at least ½ inch apart from its neighbor. Pop the ghee into the freezer for 10 minutes to chill.

Place all the dry ingredients in the bowl of a food processor and pulse a few times to mix well. Remove the ghee from the freezer, and use a butter knife to cut each tablespoon into quarters; scrape them into the food processor, and pulse until the mixture resembles moist sand. Add the flaxseed mixture, maple syrup, and vanilla extract, and pulse again until the dough comes together and balls up slightly. Be careful not to overprocess.

Turn the dough out onto a large cutting board dusted with cassava flour. Knead briefly, just until the dough comes together, then roll it into a log 12 inches long by 2 inches in diameter. Cover the log in plastic wrap and chill in the fridge for 2 hours. (You can also refrigerate the dough for up to a week until ready to use, or double wrap and freeze up to 2 months. Thaw frozen dough for 24 hours in the refrigerator before slicing.)

Preheat the oven to 350°F, and arrange 2 racks in the center of the oven. Line 2 baking sheets with parchment paper.

Makes about 4 dozen biscuits

2 tablespoons flaxseed meal or ground flaxseed

5 tablespoons hot water

8 tablespoons room-temperature ghee

1 cup superfine blanched almond flour

1¼ cups cassava flour (such as Otto's), plus more for dusting

1 teaspoon kosher sea salt

⅓ cup maple syrup

1 tablespoon alcohol-free vanilla extract

Remove the dough log from the fridge, cut into ¼-inch-thick slices, and arrange on the prepared sheets, evenly spaced. (They won't expand much.) Bake for 18 minutes, or until fragrant and lightly golden brown at the edges.

Remove from the oven and allow to cool completely, about an hour. Store in an airtight container at room temperature for up to a week.

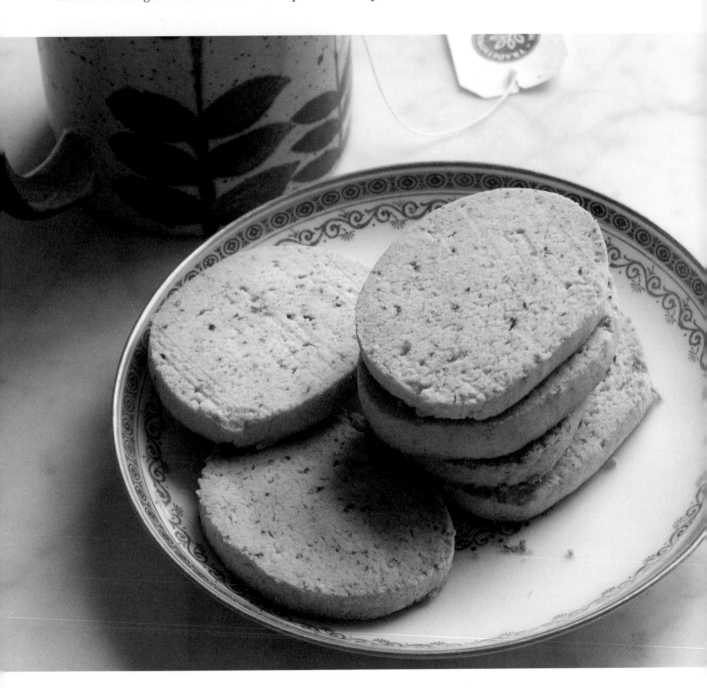

Date + Cacao Truffles

Truth be told, I'm not a huge dessert person. I absolutely love a slice of birthday cake and an ice-cream cup in the summer, but mostly I'm looking for a small, sweet ending to my meals, preferably strong dark chocolate. If I owned a restaurant, I would serve an assortment of chocolate bars wrapped in beautiful paper and an assortment of homemade truffles on a silver platter. These are tiny, intensely rich, and coated in powerful ingredients, too, making them an upgrade to any dessert fantasy. They are also lovely to serve at a dinner party.

I like using multiple coatings for my truffles, but for simplicity, you can choose just one if you prefer. My personal favorites are hemp seeds, bee pollen, and cacao powder, but try other coatings like shredded coconut, ground pistachios and other nuts, berry powders, or sesame seeds.

Line a small baking sheet with parchment paper.

Fill 3 small bowls with each of the coatings: hemp seeds, bee pollen, and cacao powder.

In the bowl of a food processor, pulse the dates about 30 times, until broken down. Add the cacao powder, coconut butter, coconut oil, vanilla extract, and salt. Pulse again a few times, until the dough balls up. Using a small scoop or spoon, measure a 2-teaspoon-size portion of the dough and roll it into a ball between your hands. If the dough sticks, you can wet your hands with a little water. Repeat with the remaining dough, placing the balls onto the prepared baking sheet as you work.

Roll each ball again in one of the coatings, so you have a roughly even number of coated truffles. Return each truffle to the baking sheet as you work. Refrigerate until firm, about 2 hours. You can serve them immediately, or store them in an airtight container in the fridge for up to 3 weeks.

Makes 14 truffles

¼ cup hemp seeds, for coating

¼ cup bee pollen, for coating

½ cup cacao powder, plus ¼ cup for coating

14 Medjool dates, pitted

2 tablespoons coconut butter, melted

2 tablespoons coconut oil

1 tablespoon alcohol-free vanilla extract

Pinch of kosher sea salt

Tips
You can also freeze the truffles—just place the dish of completed truffles in the freezer for 4 hours, until frozen solid, then transfer to an airtight container and store for up to 6 months.

Coconut butter can be found either near the coconut oil in the oil section of a supermarket or with other nut butters.

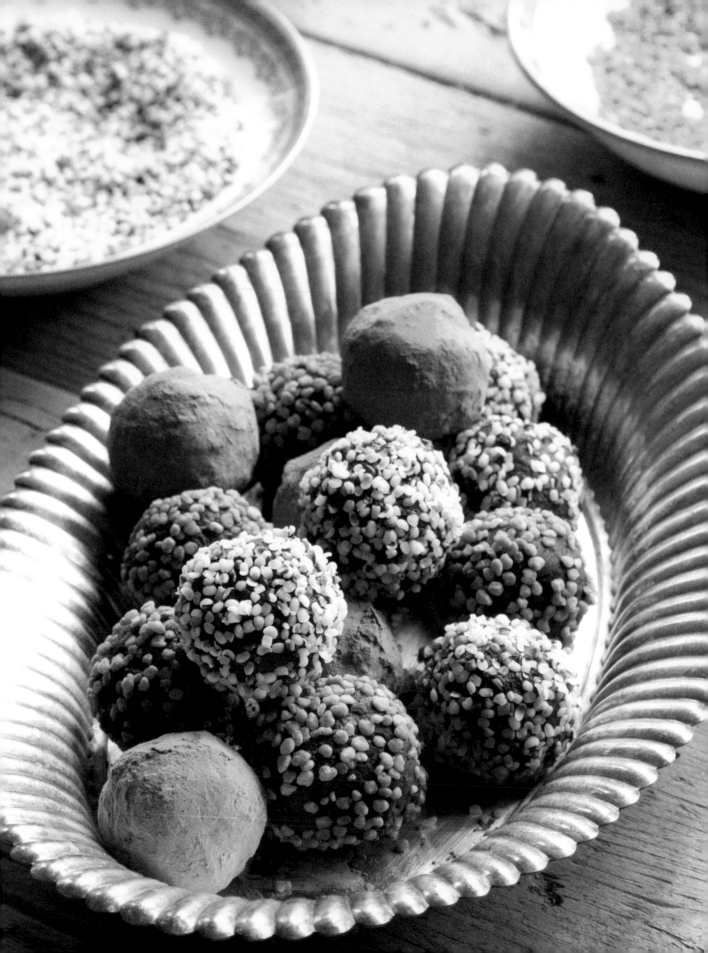

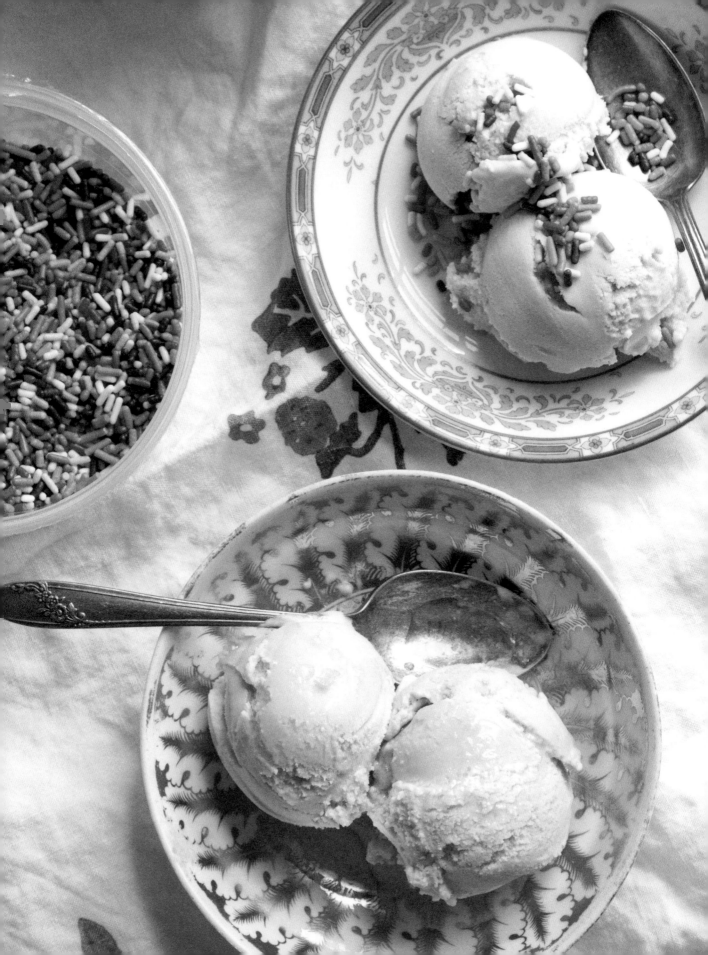

Vanilla Ice Cream

I still love vanilla ice cream with rainbow sprinkles like I did when I was eight years old. We used to live across the street from Häagen-Dazs, and my father would take me there once a week for a treat. I ordered the same thing every time; I still do. Since I gave up dairy, I've been fanatical about finding great dairy-free substitutes, which can be hard because they are usually loaded with all sorts of unhealthy ingredients. I've developed this recipe so I can eat my favorite ice cream with abandon. The key to success with making a dairy-free coconut cream–based ice cream is that you need to heat up the mixture first, blend it, and then cool it before freezing. You'll also need to use regular vanilla extract—not alcohol-free. There's some vital chemistry in these steps and ingredients that works. It does take a little planning (you'll need to start the ice cream at least 12 hours before you want to serve it), but the results are so worth it. Make sure your coconut cream has no gums or fillers. We need full-fat, all-natural cream.

Put the tub of an ice-cream maker into the freezer the day before you plan to make the ice cream and let it freeze for a full 24 hours before using.

Makes about 1 quart

2 (13.5-ounce) cans heavy coconut cream (such as from Let's Do Organic or Nature's Greatest Foods)

½ cup maple syrup

¼ cup coconut oil

¼ teaspoon kosher sea salt

1 tablespoon vanilla extract (not alcohol-free)

Sauce It
Serve with Vanilla Berry Compote (page 32) or Caramel Sauce (page 211), top with rainbow sprinkles, or simply drizzle with extra-virgin olive oil and a sprinkle of flaky sea salt.

In a medium saucepan, combine the coconut cream, maple syrup, coconut oil, and salt, and simmer, whisking constantly for about 2 minutes. Transfer the mixture to an upright blender and blend on high for 30 seconds. Transfer to a container with a lid, allow to cool uncovered for 30 minutes, then stir in the vanilla extract. Cover and place in the fridge to chill for 4 hours, or overnight.

Once chilled, give the mixture a quick whisk again to blend in the skin of fat and any separation that may have formed while in the fridge. Transfer to an ice-cream maker and churn according to the manufacturer's instructions. At this point, the ice cream will resemble soft serve. You can enjoy it immediately, or transfer it to a freezer-safe container with a lid to firm up more in the freezer, another 3 to 4 hours, or overnight.

To serve, remove the ice cream from the freezer and allow to reach room temperature, about 15 minutes, or until soft enough to scoop.

Resources

Below is a list of some of my favorite books, pantry items, and kitchen tools. All of them have supported my health journey in some way and have helped me get delicious meals on the table.

I have also included a list of doctors I have seen personally as a patient or whose work I have followed very closely. They all have a root-cause approach to medicine.

Books

The Autoimmune Paleo Cookbook
Mickey Trescott, NTP

Hashimoto's Thyroiditis
Izabella Wentz, PharmD, FASCP

Thyroid Healthy
Suzy Cohen, RPh

Anatomy of the Spirit
Caroline Myss

Pantry Items

Bob's Red Mill / bobsredmill.com

Otto's Naturals / ottosnaturals.com

Jovial Foods / jovialfoods.com

Zona Food Market / zonafoodmarket.com

Kitchen Tools

Instant Pot / instanthome.com

Cuisinart / cuisinart.com

Vitamix / vitamix.com

KitchenAid / kitchenaid.com

Lodge / lodgecastiron.com

Le Creuset / lecreuset.com

Doctors

Dr. Steven Bock / bockmd.com

Dr. Will Cole / drwillcole.com

Dr. Sara Gottfried / saragottfriedmd.com

Dr. Daniel Amen / amenclinics.com

Dr. Frank Lipman / drfranklipman.com

Dr. Mark Hyman / drhyman.com

Dr. Ben Lynch / drbenlynch.com

Dr. Josh Axe / draxe.com

Acknowledgments

First and foremost, thank you to my husband, Mark. My journey back to health would have been impossible without your patient and unwavering love and support. You have had faith in my recovery and creativity from the start—I could not have done any of it without you. And thank you for tasting fish sauce and chocolate cake at 8:00 a.m., when I seemed to need your input most. To our girls, Jane and Rose, thank you for always cheering me on and telling it like it is. Thank you for helping me take pictures and for pulling it all together in the final hours. I love you all more than you know.

To Kate MacKinnon, your guidance, mentorship, and generosity have felt divine to me since the moment we met. Thank you for introducing me to LeAnna Weller Smith. LeAnna, thank you for bringing my blog to life and for connecting me with publicist Andrea Burnett. Andrea, thank you for your enthusiasm and for recognizing I needed to start my book journey with Leslie Jonath.

Leslie, thank you for taking me on. Working on the proposal with you was a turning point. I learned so much. Your expertise, kindness, and faith in my work gave me the courage to keep going. Thank you for agenting this book, having my back, and finding the *perfect* home for it at Girl Friday Productions.

To my publisher, Kristin Mehus-Roe, thank you for seeing and believing in my vision so clearly. To my publishing manager, Emilie Sandoz-Voyer, thank you for the many brainstorming sessions, being a fantastic and supportive sounding board, answering the same questions over and over, and having patience with me and my many Zoom challenges.

To Jess Thomson, you are the most badass developmental editor and recipe tester around. You taught me how to write real recipes. You helped me find my voice. You held me accountable. You made me laugh. You got me to the finish line. Thank you for all of it, truly.

A very big thank-you to designer Debbie Berne, art director Paul Barrett, publishing manager Kristin Duran, production editor Abi Pollokoff, copyeditor Carrie Wicks, marketing strategist Adria Batt, publishing coordinator Aidan Davis, proofreader Brittany Dowdle, and the entire team at Girl Friday Productions. What an incredible and empowering experience it was to create my first book with you all.

Thank you to Erica Goldsmith for helping me recipe test that tricky grain-free boule. Thank you to all of my daughters' teenage friends who gave me the brutal honesty I needed in order to make my bread and cake dreams come true.

A special thank-you to my assistant, Deandra Edwards. You were a lifesaver—with your positivity, warmth, organizational superpowers, and the ability to wear all the hats and find time when I needed you most, with a smile on your face. You are the best.

To my parents, granny Merle, and my dearest family and friends across the globe who continue to support me and cheer me on from the sidelines and the heavens: I love you so, so much.

Lastly, I would like to give a special thanks to my precious body—we've been through a lot together. I can always count on you to tell me the truth and to heal if I listen.

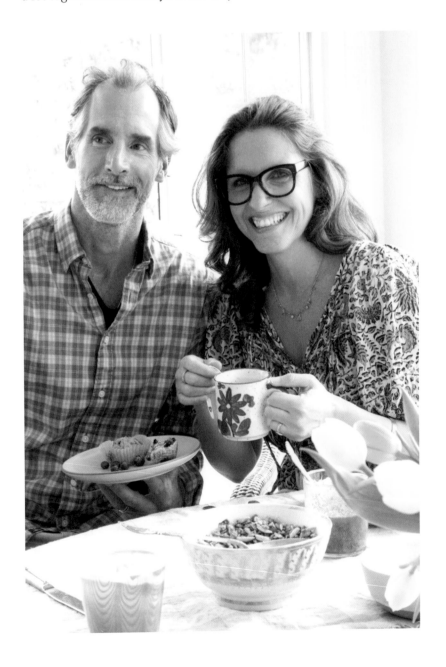

Index

aioli. *See* Chipotle Aioli
almond butter
    about, xiv
    Creamy Thai Pesto, 11
almond cream, xvi. *See also* Fresh
    Almond Cream
almond flour
    about, xv
    Caramel Pear Galette, 211–13
    Carrot Birthday Cake, 217–18
    Fluffy Silver Dollar Pancakes, 57
    Grain-Free Dark Chocolate Cake,
        215–16
    Grain-Free Granola, 54
    Grain-Free Vegan Boule, 201–2
    Heirloom Tomato Galette, 209–10
    Nut + Seed Bread, 205
    Shortbread Tea Biscuits, 220–21
    Wild Blueberry Muffins, 58
almond milk
    about, xv
    Creamy Overnight Seed Pudding,
        53
    Fluffy Silver Dollar Pancakes, 57
    Grain-Free Dark Chocolate Cake,
        215–16
    Super Green Veg + Fruit Shake, 50
    Wild Blueberry Muffins, 58
almonds
    Black Friday Korma, 100
    Chipotle Aioli, 21
    Fresh Almond Cream, 16
    Fresh Almond Ricotta Cheese, 15,
        32
    Grain-Free Granola, 54
anchovies
    Caesar Dressing, 9
    Turnip Green Pesto, 127
    Whole-Lemon Anchovy Dressing, 9
Anjou pears, Caramel Pear Galette,
    211–13
apples, Curried Wild Tuna Salad, xviii,
    82
arrowroot flour
    about, xv
    Caramel Pear Galette, 211–13
    Fluffy Silver Dollar Pancakes, 57
    Grain-Free Vegan Boule, 201–2
    Heirloom Tomato Galette, 209–10
    Wild Blueberry Muffins, 58
arugula
    Mandarin, Avocado + Watercress
        Salad, 81
    Tinned Fish Breakfast Salad, 65
avocado oil
    about, xiv

Carrot Birthday Cake, 217–18
Grain-Free Dark Chocolate Cake,
    215–16
Wild Blueberry Muffins, 58
avocado-oil mayonnaise, Remoulade
    Sauce, 155
avocados
    Caesar Salad with Avocado,
        Croutons + Hemp Seeds 73
    Chicory Chop Salad, 77
    House Pesto, 10
    Mandarin, Avocado + Watercress
        Salad, 81
    Smashed Cumin Guacamole, 22
    Tinned Fish Breakfast Salad, 65
Awase Dashi, 92

baby back ribs, Slow-Roasted, with
    Sticky Plum BBQ Sauce, 182
bacon
    Chicory Chop Salad, 77
    Heirloom Tomato Salad, 78
    Maple Bacon + Veg, 61
bananas
    Fluffy Silver Dollar Pancakes, 57
    Super Green Veg + Fruit Shake, 50
basil
    Cherry Tomato Confit, 18
    Creamy Thai Pesto, 11
    House Pesto, 10
    Tagliatelle Bolognese, 110
BBQ sauce, Sticky Plum, 26
bean sprouts, Creamy Pad Thai Kelp
    Noodles, 117
beans. *See also* green beans
    about, xix
    Beans, Greens + Broken Eggs, 62
    Big Batch of Beans, 40–41
    Cauliflower Cannellini Bean Mash,
        130
    White Bean + Chorizo Stew, 99
bee pollen
    Date + Cacao Truffles, 222
    Super Green Veg + Fruit Shake, 50
beef. *See also* bone broth
    Eggplant Moussaka Bake with Fresh
        Almond Ricotta, 114–15
    Grilled Skirt Steak with House
        Chimichurri, 181
    Middle Eastern Spiced Ground
        Bison, 178
    Tagliatelle Bolognese, 110
Bibb lettuce. *See* lettuce
Big Batch of Beans, 40–41
Big Batch of Short-Grain Rice, 44–45

bison, Middle Eastern Spiced Ground,
    178
Black Friday Korma, 100
black pepper, about, xvii
blueberries
    Fluffy Silver Dollar Pancakes, 57
    Wild Blueberry Muffins, 58
bone broth
    Bone Broth, 38
    Bone Broth Vegetable Purée, 88
    Red Lentil Mulligatawny Soup, 95
    White Bean + Chorizo Stew, 99
Bone Broth, 38
Bone Broth Vegetable Purée, 88
bonito flakes, Awase Dashi, 92
Boston lettuce. *See* lettuce
branzino, Whole Roasted, 151
bread, baking + sweets, 190–225
    Caramel Pear Galette, 211–13
    Carrot Birthday Cake with
        Cultured Buttercream + Rainbow
        Sprinkles, 217–18
    Cassava Tortillas, 197–98
    Cheesy Garlic Croutons, 12
    Date + Cacao Truffles, 222
    Flatbreads, 194
    Grain-Free Dark Chocolate Cake
        with Chocolate Sweet Potato
        Frosting, 215–16
    Grain-Free Vegan Boule, 201–2
    Heirloom Tomato Galette, 209–10
    Nut + Seed Bread, 205
    Shortbread Tea Biscuits, 220–21
    Sweet Potato Tortillas, 197–98
    Tortillas, 197–98
    Vanilla Ice Cream, 225
    Wild Blueberry Muffins, 58
breakfast. *See* mornings
broccoli
    Bone Broth Vegetable Purée, 88
    Non-Starchy Roasted Vegetables,
        123
    "rice," 123
broccoli rabe, Garlicky Greens with
    Apple Cider Vinegar, 131
Broccolini, Garlicky Greens with
    Apple Cider Vinegar, 131
broth. *See* bone broth
brown rice, Short-Grain, 45
brown rice spaghetti, Lemon
    Spaghetti, 109
Brussels sprouts, Crispy, with Fish
    Sauce Caramel, 124
butter. *See* almond butter; coconut
    butter; ghee

butter lettuce. *See* lettuce
butternut squash, Bone Broth
 Vegetable Purée, 88

cabbage
 Creamy Pad Thai Kelp Noodles, 117
 Quick Pickled Slaw, 156
cacao powder
 about, xv
 Date + Cacao Truffles, 222
 Grain-Free Dark Chocolate Cake
  with Chocolate Sweet Potato
  Frosting, 215–16
Cacio e Pepe 2.0, 113
Caesar Dressing, 9, 73
Caesar Salad with Avocado, Croutons +
 Hemp Seeds, 73
cake
 Carrot Birthday Cake with
  Cultured Buttercream + Rainbow
  Sprinkles, 217–18
 Grain-Free Dark Chocolate Cake
  with Chocolate Sweet Potato
  Frosting, 215–16
canned beans. *See* beans
cannellini beans
 Cauliflower Cannellini Bean Mash,
  130
 White Bean + Chorizo Stew, 99
Caper-Currant Relish, 25, 128
capers
 about, xviii
 Green Onion Salsa, 6
 Caper-Currant Relish, 25
Caramel Pear Galette, 211–13
Caramel Sauce, 211
Carnitas, 185
Carrot Birthday Cake with Cultured
 Buttercream + Rainbow
 Sprinkles, 217–18
carrots
 Carrot Birthday Cake with
  Cultured Buttercream + Rainbow
  Sprinkles, 217–18
 Creamy Pad Thai Kelp Noodles, 117
 Red Lentil Mulligatawny Soup, 95
 Rotisserie Chicken Soup, 91
cassava flour
 about, xv
 Carrot Birthday Cake, 217–18
 Cassava Tortillas, 197–98
 Flatbreads, 194
 Flounder Meunière, 160
 Fried Oysters with Remoulade
  Sauce, 155
 Grain-Free Dark Chocolate Cake,
  215–16
 Shortbread Tea Biscuits, 220–21
 Sweet Potato Tortillas, 197–98

Wild Fried Fish Tacos, 156–57
Cassava Tortillas, 197–98
 Carnitas, 185
 Wild Fried Fish Tacos with Quick
  Pickled Slaw + Chipotle Aioli,
  156–57
cauliflower
 Cauliflower Cannellini Bean Mash,
  130
 Crispy Brussels Sprouts with Fish
  Sauce Caramel, 124
 Maple Bacon + Veg, 61
 Non-Starchy Roasted Vegetables,
  123
 Pan-Roasted Cauliflower with
  Caper-Currant Relish + Yogurt-
  Tahini Sauce, 128
 "rice," 123
Cauliflower Cannellini Bean Mash, 130
chard. *See* greens
cheese. *See also* nutritional yeast
 Cheesy Garlic Croutons, 12
 Fresh Almond Ricotta Cheese, 15
 Tagliatelle Bolognese, 110
Cheesy Garlic Croutons, 12
 Caesar Salad with Avocado,
  Croutons + Hemp Seeds, 73
cherry tomatoes
 Cherry Tomato Confit, 18
 Penne alla Rosé, 106
chia seeds
 Creamy Overnight Seed Pudding,
  53
 Nut + Seed Bread, 205
chicken. *See also* bone broth
 Black Friday Korma, 100
 Chicken Liver Pâté, 169
 Chicken Thighs with Green Olives,
  Dates, Lemon + Butter Lettuce,
  173
 Gochujang Wings, 166–67
 Mandarin, Avocado + Watercress
  Salad, 81
 Overnight Roast Chicken, 174
 "Sour Cream" + Onion Chicken
  Thigh Schnitzel with Chip
  Crumbs, 170–71
chickpeas, Curried Wild Tuna Salad, 82
Chicory Chop Salad, 77
chimichurri, House, 5
Chipotle Aioli, 21
chocolate. *see* cacao powder
chorizo, Stew, White Bean +, 99
chutney, Cilantro-Mint, 7
cilantro
 Black Friday Korma, 100
 Cilantro-Mint Chutney, 7
 Clams with Ginger-Coconut Broth,
  96
 Quick Pickled Slaw, 156

Red Lentil Mulligatawny Soup, 95
 Smashed Cumin Guacamole, 22
 Tinned Fish Breakfast Salad, 65
Citrus-Cured Lox, 145–46
Clams with Ginger-Coconut Broth, 96
coconut, shredded
 Creamy Overnight Seed Pudding,
  53
 Wild Blueberry Muffins, 58
coconut aminos, xviii
coconut butter
 about, xiv
 Cultured Buttercream, 218
coconut cream
 about, xvi
 Vanilla Ice Cream, 225
coconut flour
 about, xv
 Carrot Birthday Cake, 217–18
 Fluffy Silver Dollar Pancakes, 57
 Grain-Free Dark Chocolate Cake,
  215–16
 Wild Blueberry Muffins, 58
coconut milk
 about, xvi
 Carrot Birthday Cake, 217–18
 Clams with Ginger-Coconut Broth,
  96
coconut oil
 about, xiv
 Chocolate Sweet Potato Frosting,
  215–16
 Cultured Buttercream, 218
 Grain-Free Granola, 54
 Vanilla Ice Cream, 225
coconut sugar
 about, xvi
 Carrot Birthday Cake, 217–18
 Citrus-Cured Lox, 145–46
coconut yogurt
 about, xvi
 Black Friday Korma, 100
 Cilantro-Mint Chutney, 7
 Coconut Yogurt Tzatziki, 31
 Cultured Buttercream, 218
 Curried Wild Tuna Salad, xviii, 82
 Flatbreads, 194
 Red Lentil Mulligatawny Soup, 95
 "Sour Cream" + Onion Chicken
  Thigh Schnitzel with Chip
  Crumbs, 170–71
 Super Green Veg + Fruit Shake, 50
 Yogurt-Tahini Sauce, 128
Coconut Yogurt Tzatziki, 31
 Lamb Koftas, 189
 Turkey Zucchini Patties with
  Coconut Yogurt Tzatziki, 177
collard greens. *See* greens
Confit Three Ways, 17–18

cookies, Shortbread Tea Biscuits, 220–21
country-style Dijon mustard, xviii, 6, 8, 9, 21, 82, 155, 182, 186
cream alternatives, xvi. *See also* almond cream; coconut cream
Creamy Overnight Seed Pudding, 53
Creamy Pad Thai Kelp Noodles, 117
Creamy Thai Pesto, 11, 117
Crispy Broiled King Salmon, 148
Crispy Brussels Sprouts with Fish Sauce Caramel, 124
Crispy Oven-Fried Sweet Potatoes, 137
croutons. *See* Cheesy Garlic Croutons
cucumbers, Quick Pickled, 29
Cultured Buttercream, 218
currants
    Caper-Currant Relish, 25
    House Pesto, 10
    Tuscan Kale Salad with Pomegranate, Pine Nuts +, 74
Curried Wild Tuna Salad, 82

dairy alternatives, xv–xvi
dates
    about, xvi–xvii
    Chicken Thighs with Green Olives, Dates, Lemon + Butter Lettuce, 173
    Date + Cacao Truffles, 222
delicata squash, Starchy Roasted Vegetables, 123
desserts. *See* bread, baking + sweets
Dijon mustard, xviii
dill
    Butter Lettuce with Fresh Herbs, Toasted Maple Sunflower Seeds + Marlit's Vinaigrette, 70
    Citrus-Cured Lox, 145–46
    Coconut Yogurt Tzatziki, 31
    Rotisserie Chicken Soup, 91
    Tinned Fish Breakfast Salad, 65
dried beans. *See* beans

Eggplant Moussaka Bake with Fresh Almond Ricotta, 114–15
eggs
    Beans, Greens + Broken Eggs, 62
    Span-ish Frittata with Spinach, 138
escarole. *See* lettuce
extra-virgin olive oil, about, xiv

fennel
    Clams with Ginger-Coconut Broth, 96
fish. *See* seafood; tinned fish
fish sauce
    about, xviii

Crispy Brussels Sprouts with Fish Sauce Caramel, 124
Flatbreads, 194
flat-leaf parsley. *See* parsley
flaxseed meal
    about, xv
    Carrot Birthday Cake, 217–18
    Creamy Overnight Seed Pudding, 53
    Grain-Free Dark Chocolate Cake, 215–16
    Nut + Seed Bread, 205
    Shortbread Tea Biscuits, 220–21
    Wild Blueberry Muffins, 58
Flounder Meunière, 160
flour, grain-free, xv
Fluffy Silver Dollar Pancakes, 57
Fresh Almond Cream, 16
    Caramel Pear Galette, 211–13
    Penne alla Rosé, 106
    Red Lentil Mulligatawny Soup, 95
Fresh Almond Ricotta Cheese, 15
    Eggplant Moussaka Bake with, 114–15
    Heirloom Tomato Galette, 209–10
    Vanilla Berry Compote, 32
Fried Oysters with Remoulade Sauce, 155
frisée. *See* lettuce
fruit, Shake, Super Green Veg +, 50

galettes
    Caramel Pear Galette, 211–13
    Heirloom Tomato Galette, 209–10
Garlic Confit, 18
    Cauliflower Cannellini Bean Mash, 130
garlic croutons, Cheesy, 12
    Caesar Salad with Avocado, Croutons + Hemp Seeds, 73
Garlicky Greens with Apple Cider Vinegar, 131
ghee, about, xiv
ginger-coconut broth, Clams with, 96
gluten-free flours + binders, xv
gluten-free pasta. *See* pasta + noodles
Gochujang Wings, 166–67
Grain-Free Dark Chocolate Cake with Chocolate Sweet Potato Frosting, 215–16
Grain-Free Granola, 54
Grain-Free Vegan Boule, 201–2
    Cheesy Garlic Croutons, 12, 73
    White Bean + Chorizo Stew, 99
granola, Grain-Free, 54
Grass-Fed Rack of Lamb, 186
Greek-style coconut yogurt. *See* coconut yogurt
green olives. *See* olives

green onions
    Clams with Ginger-Coconut Broth, 96
    Creamy Pad Thai Kelp Noodles, 117
    Green Onion Salsa, 6
greens
    Awase Dashi, 92
    Beans, Greens + Broken Eggs, 62
    Bone Broth Vegetable Purée, 88
    Eggplant Moussaka Bake with Fresh Almond Ricotta, 114–15
    Garlicky Greens with Apple Cider Vinegar, 131
    Mandarin, Avocado + Watercress Salad, 81
    Rotisserie Chicken Soup, 91
    Span-ish Frittata with Spinach, 138
    Super Green Veg + Fruit Shake, 50
    Tinned Fish Breakfast Salad, 65
    Tuscan Kale Salad with Pomegranate, Pine Nuts + Currants, 74
    White Bean + Chorizo Stew, 99
Grilled Skirt Steak with House Chimichurri, 181
ground flaxseed. *See* flaxseed meal
guacamole, Smashed Cumin, 22

Heirloom Tomato Galette, 209–10
Heirloom Tomato Salad, 78
hemp seeds
    Caesar Salad with Avocado, Croutons +, 73
    Date + Cacao Truffles, 222
honey, xvi
    Quick Pickles, 28–29
    Honeycrisp apples, Curried Wild Tuna Salad, 82
honeynut squash, Roasted, 133
House Chimichurri, 5
    Grilled Skirt Steak with, 181
House Pesto, 10

ice cream, Vanilla, 225
Italian parsley. *See* parsley
Italian-style "breading," 37

kale. *See* greens
kelp noodles, Creamy Pad Thai, 117
koftas, Lamb, 189
kombu, Awase Dashi, 92
korma, Black Friday, 100
kosher sea salt, xvii

Lacinato kale. *See* greens
lamb. *See also* bone broth
    Black Friday Korma, 100
    Eggplant Moussaka Bake with Fresh Almond Ricotta, 114–15

Grass-Fed Rack of Lamb, 186
Lamb Koftas, 189
White Bean + Chorizo Stew, 99
lemon
Caesar Dressing, 9
Lemon Spaghetti, 109
"Sour Cream" + Onion Chicken
Thigh Schnitzel with Chip
Crumbs, 170–71
Whole-Lemon Anchovy Dressing, 9
lentils, Red, Mulligatawny Soup, 95
lettuce
Butter Lettuce with Fresh Herbs,
Toasted Maple Sunflower Seeds +
Marlit's Vinaigrette, 70
Caesar Salad with Avocado,
Croutons + Hemp Seeds, 73
Chicken Thighs with Green Olives,
Dates, Lemon + Butter Lettuce,
173
Chicory Chop Salad, 77
Tinned Fish Breakfast Salad, 65
lox, Citrus-Cured, 145–46

Mandarin, Avocado + Watercress
Salad, 81
Maple Bacon + Veg, 61
maple syrup
about, xvi
Caramel Sauce, 211
Carrot Birthday Cake with
Cultured Buttercream + Rainbow
Sprinkles, 217–18
Crispy Brussels Sprouts with Fish
Sauce Caramel, 124
Grain-Free Dark Chocolate Cake
with Chocolate Sweet Potato
Frosting, 215–16
Shortbread Tea Biscuits, 220–21
Toasted Maple Sunflower Seeds, 35
Vanilla Ice Cream, 225
Wild Blueberry Muffins, 58
Marlit's Vinaigrette, 8
Butter Lettuce with Fresh Herbs,
Toasted Maple Sunflower Seeds +
Marlit's Vinaigrette, 70
Heirloom Tomato Salad, 78
mayonnaise, Remoulade Sauce, 155
meatballs. See koftas
Middle Eastern Spiced Ground Bison,
178
milk alternatives. See almond milk;
coconut milk; dairy alternatives
mint
Cilantro-Mint Chutney, 7
Lamb Koftas, 189
mornings, 46–65
Beans, Greens + Broken Eggs, 62
Creamy Overnight Seed Pudding,
53

Fluffy Silver Dollar Pancakes, 57
Grain-Free Granola, 54
Maple Bacon + Veg, 61
Super Green Veg + Fruit Shake, 50
Tinned Fish Breakfast Salad, 65
Wild Blueberry Muffins, 58
moussaka bake, Eggplant, with Fresh
Almond Ricotta, 114–15
muffins, Wild Blueberry, 58
mulligatawny soup, Red Lentil, 95
mushrooms
Awase Dashi, 92
Wild Mushrooms with Ghee, Herbs
+ Sherry Vinegar, 134
mustard. See country-style Dijon
mustard
mustard greens. See greens

nightshades, xii
Non-Starchy Roasted Vegetables, 123
noodles. See pasta + noodles
Nut + Seed Bread, 205
nutritional yeast
about, xvii
Cacio e Pepe 2.0, 113
Caesar Dressing, 9
Cauliflower Cannellini Bean Mash,
130
Cheesy Garlic Croutons, 12
Heirloom Tomato Galette, 209–10
House Pesto, 10
Lemon Spaghetti, 109
nuts. See also seeds
Black Friday Korma, 100
Caper-Currant Relish, 25
Carrot Birthday Cake, 217–18
Chicory Chop Salad, 77
Chipotle Aioli, 21
Fresh Almond Cream, 16
Fresh Almond Ricotta Cheese, 15
Grain-Free Granola, 54
House Pesto, 10
Nut + Seed Bread, 205
Turnip Green Pesto, 127
Tuscan Kale Salad with
Pomegranate, Pine Nuts +
Currants, 74

olive oil. See extra-virgin olive oil
olives
about, xviii
Chicken Thighs with Green Olives,
Dates, Lemon + Butter Lettuce,
173
Overnight Roast Chicken, 174
Rotisserie Chicken Soup, 91
oysters, Fried, with Remoulade Sauce,
155

pad thai, Creamy, Kelp Noodles, 117
pancakes, Fluffy Silver Dollar, 57
Pan-Roasted Cauliflower with Caper-
Currant Relish + Yogurt-Tahini
Sauce, 128
Pan-Sautéed Baby Turnips with Turnip
Green Pesto, 127
parsley
Chicory Chop Salad, 77
Green Onion Salsa, 6
House Chimichurri, 5
Lamb Koftas, 189
Lemon Spaghetti, 109
Rotisserie Chicken Soup, 91
Turkey Zucchini Patties with
Coconut Yogurt Tzatziki, 177
Wild Mushrooms with Ghee, Herbs
+ Sherry Vinegar, 134
pasta + noodles, 102–17
alternative grains, about, xiii, xix
Cacio e Pepe 2.0, 113
Creamy Pad Thai Kelp Noodles, 117
Eggplant Moussaka Bake with Fresh
Almond Ricotta, 114–15
Lemon Spaghetti, 109
Penne alla Rosé, 106
Tagliatelle Bolognese, 110
peanut butter, Creamy Thai Pesto, 11
pear, Caramel Pear Galette, 211–13
Penne alla Rosé, 106
pepitas. See pumpkin seeds
pesto
Creamy Thai Pesto, 11, 117
House Pesto, 10
Turnip Green Pesto, 127
pickles, Quick, 28–29
pies. See galettes
pine nuts
Caper-Currant Relish, 25
House Pesto, 10
Turnip Green Pesto, 127
Tuscan Kale Salad with
Pomegranate, Pine Nuts +
Currants, 74
plantain chips
"Sour Cream" + Onion Chicken
Thigh Schnitzel with Chip
Crumbs, 170–71
Toasted Plantain Crumbs, 37
plum, Sticky, BBQ Sauce, 26
pomegranate
Pan-Roasted Cauliflower with
Caper-Currant Relish + Yogurt-
Tahini Sauce, 128
Tuscan Kale Salad with
Pomegranate, Pine Nuts +
Currants, 74
pork. See also bone broth
Carnitas, 185

pork *continued*
    Slow-Roasted Ribs with Sticky Plum BBQ Sauce, 182
    White Bean + Chorizo Stew, 99
potatoes, Span-ish Frittata with Spinach, 138
prawns, Whole Garlic, with Charred Lemon, 159
psyllium husk
    about, xv
    Grain-Free Vegan Boule, 201–2
    Nut + Seed Bread, 205
    Wild Blueberry Muffins, 58
pudding, Creamy Overnight Seed, 53
pumpkin seeds
    Grain-Free Granola, 54
    House Pesto, 10
    Nut + Seed Bread, 205
    Pan-Sautéed Baby Turnips with Turnip Green Pesto, 127
    Za'atar Toasted Pepitas, 34
purple cabbage. *See* cabbage

Quick Pickled Cucumbers, 29
Quick Pickled Radishes, 28
Quick Pickled Red Onions, 28
Quick Pickled Slaw, 156
Quick Pickles, 28–29
quinoa, Nut + Seed Bread, 205

radicchio
    Chicory Chop Salad, 77
    Tinned Fish Breakfast Salad, 65
radishes
    Quick Pickled Radishes, 28
    Tinned Fish Breakfast Salad, 65
rainbow chard. *See* greens
Red Lentil Mulligatawny Soup, 95
red onions, Quick Pickled, 28
remoulade sauce, Fried Oysters with, 155
ribs, Slow-Roasted, with Sticky Plum BBQ Sauce, 182
rice
    about, xix
    Big Batch of Short-Grain Rice, 44–45
    broccoli or cauliflower "rice," 123
    Clams with Ginger-Coconut Broth, 96
    Short-Grain Brown Rice, 45
    Sushi Rice, 45
Roasted Honeynut Squash, 133
roasted vegetables
    Non-Starchy, 123
    Starchy, 123
    Steak Knife, 122–23
romaine lettuce. *See* lettuce
Rotisserie Chicken Soup, 91

salads + small plates, 66–83
    Butter Lettuce with Fresh Herbs, Toasted Maple Sunflower Seeds + Marlit's Vinaigrette, 70
    Caesar Salad with Avocado, Croutons + Hemp Seeds, 73
    Chicory Chop Salad, 77
    Curried Wild Tuna Salad, 82
    Heirloom Tomato Salad, 78
    Mandarin, Avocado + Watercress Salad, 81
    Three Dressings, 8–9
    Tinned Fish Breakfast Salad, 65
    Tuscan Kale Salad with Pomegranate, Pine Nuts + Currants, 74
salmon
    Citrus-Cured Lox, 145–46
    Crispy Broiled King Salmon, 148
salsa, Green Onion, 6
salt, about, xvii
sardines. *See* tinned fish
sauces + staples, 1–45
    about, xiii
    Big Batch of Beans, 40–41
    Big Batch of Short-Grain Rice, 44–45
    Bone Broth, 38
    Caesar Dressing, 9
    Caper-Currant Relish, 25
    Cheesy Garlic Croutons, 12
    Cherry Tomato Confit, 18
    Chipotle Aioli, 21
    Cilantro-Mint Chutney, 7
    Coconut Yogurt Tzatziki, 31
    Confit Three Ways, 17–18
    Creamy Thai Pesto, 11
    Fresh Almond Cream, 16
    Fresh Almond Ricotta Cheese, 15
    Garlic Confit, 18
    Green Onion Salsa, 6
    House Chimichurri, 5
    House Pesto, 10
    Marlit's Vinaigrette, 8
    Quick Pickled Cucumbers, 29
    Quick Pickled Radishes, 28
    Quick Pickled Red Onions, 28
    Quick Pickles, 28–29
    Shallot Confit, 17
    Short-Grain Brown Rice, 45
    Smashed Cumin Guacamole, 22
    Spiced Toasted Seeds, 34–35
    Sticky Plum BBQ Sauce, 26
    Sushi Rice, 45
    Three Dressings, 8–9
    Toasted Maple Sunflower Seeds, 35
    Toasted Plantain Crumbs, 37
    Vanilla Berry Compote, 32
    Whole-Lemon Anchovy Dressing, 9
    Za'atar Toasted Pepitas, 34

scallops, Seared, with Garlic Ghee, 152
seafood, 140–61. *See also* tinned fish
    Awase Dashi, 92
    Citrus-Cured Lox, 145–46
    Creamy Thai Pesto, 11
    Crispy Broiled King Salmon, 148
    Curried Wild Tuna Salad, xviii, 82
    Flounder Meunière, 160
    Fried Oysters with Remoulade Sauce, 155
    Seared Scallops with Garlic Ghee, 152
    Whole Garlic Prawns with Charred Lemon, 159
    Whole Roasted Branzino, 151
    Whole-Lemon Anchovy Dressing, 9
    Wild Fried Fish Tacos with Quick Pickled Slaw + Chipotle Aioli, 156–57
Seared Scallops with Garlic Ghee, 152
seasoning + spices, xvii
seeds. *See also* nuts
    Caesar Salad with Avocado, Croutons + Hemp Seeds, 73
    Creamy Overnight Seed Pudding, 53
    Grain-Free Granola, 54
    Spiced Toasted Seeds, 34–35
    Toasted Maple Sunflower Seeds, 35, 70
    Za'atar Toasted Pepitas, 34
shake, Super Green Veg + Fruit, 50
shallots
    Chicken Liver Pâté, 169
    Clams with Ginger-Coconut Broth, 96
    Fried Oysters with Remoulade Sauce, 155
    Shallot Confit, 17
Shortbread Tea Biscuits, 220–21
short-grain rice. *See* rice
silver dollar pancakes, Fluffy, 57
skirt steak, Grilled, with House Chimichurri, 181
Slow-Roasted Ribs with Sticky Plum BBQ Sauce, 182
Smashed Cumin Guacamole, 22
sole meunière, 160
soups + stews, 84–101
    Awase Dashi, 92
    Black Friday Korma, 100
    Bone Broth, 38
    Bone Broth Vegetable Purée, 88
    Clams with Ginger-Coconut Broth, 96
    Red Lentil Mulligatawny Soup, 95
    Rotisserie Chicken Soup, 91
    White Bean + Chorizo Stew, 99

"Sour Cream" + Onion Chicken Thigh Schnitzel with Chip Crumbs, 170–71
soy substitutes, 26
spaghetti, Lemon, 109
Span-ish Frittata with Spinach, 138
Spiced Toasted Seeds, 34–35
spices, about, xvii
spinach. *See* greens
squash
    Bone Broth Vegetable Purée, 88
    Cacio e Pepe 2.0, 113
    Roasted Honeynut Squash, 133
    Rotisserie Chicken Soup, 91
    Starchy Roasted Vegetables, 123
Starchy Roasted Vegetables, 123
Steak Knife Roasted Vegetables, 122–23
Sticky Plum BBQ Sauce, 26
    Slow-Roasted Ribs with, 182
strawberries, Vanilla Berry Compote, 32
sugar substitutes, xvi–xvii
sunflower seeds
    Grain-Free Granola, 54
    Nut + Seed Bread, 205
    Toasted Maple Sunflower Seeds, 35
Super Green Veg + Fruit Shake, 50
superfine almond flour. *See* almond flour
Sushi Rice, 45
Sweet Potato Tortillas, 197–98
sweet potatoes
    Crispy Oven-Fried Sweet Potatoes, 137
    Grain-Free Dark Chocolate Cake with Chocolate Sweet Potato Frosting, 215–16
    Red Lentil Mulligatawny Soup, 95
    Starchy Roasted Vegetables, 123
    Sweet Potato Tortillas, 197–98
sweeteners, xvi–xvii
Swiss chard. *See* greens

tacos, Wild Fried Fish, with Quick Pickled Slaw + Chipotle Aioli, 156–57
Tagliatelle Bolognese, 110
Tahini-Yogurt Sauce, 128
tamari, xviii
tapioca flour
    about, xv
    Fried Oysters with Remoulade Sauce, 155
    Grain-Free Dark Chocolate Cake, 215–16
    Wild Fried Fish Tacos, 156–57
Three Dressings, 8–9
tinned fish

about, xviii
    Caesar Dressing, 9
    Pan-Sautéed Baby Turnips with Turnip Green Pesto, 127
    Tinned Fish Breakfast Salad, 65
    Whole-Lemon Anchovy Dressing, 9
Toasted Maple Sunflower Seeds, 35
    Butter Lettuce with Fresh Herbs, Toasted Maple Sunflower Seeds + Marlit's Vinaigrette, 70
    Creamy Pad Thai Kelp Noodles, 117
Toasted Plantain Crumbs, 37
    Cacio e Pepe 2.0, 113
tomato paste, about, xviii
tomatoes
    Cherry Tomato Confit, 18
    Eggplant Moussaka Bake with Fresh Almond Ricotta, 114–15
    Heirloom Tomato Galette, 209–10
    Heirloom Tomato Salad, 78
    Penne alla Rosé, 106
    Tagliatelle Bolognese, 110
Tortillas, 197–98
    Carnitas, 185
    Wild Fried Fish Tacos with Quick Pickled Slaw + Chipotle Aioli, 156–57
truffles, Date + Cacao, 222
tuna
    about, xviii
    Curried Wild Tuna Salad, 82
    Tinned Fish Breakfast Salad, 65
turkey
    Black Friday Korma, 100
    Turkey Zucchini Patties with Coconut Yogurt Tzatziki, 177
    White Bean + Chorizo Stew, 99
turnips, baby, Pan-Sautéed, with Turnip Green Pesto, 127
Tuscan Kale Salad with Pomegranate, Pine Nuts + Currants, 74
tzatziki. *See* Coconut Yogurt Tzatziki

Vanilla Berry Compote, 32
    Fluffy Silver Dollar Pancakes, 57
    Vanilla Ice Cream, 225
    Wild Blueberry Muffins, 58
vanilla extract, about, xvii
Vanilla Ice Cream, 225
vegetables, 118–39. *See also* salads + small plates
    Cauliflower Cannellini Bean Mash, 130
    Crispy Brussels Sprouts with Fish Sauce Caramel, 124
    Crispy Oven-Fried Sweet Potatoes, 137
    Garlicky Greens with Apple Cider Vinegar, 131

Maple Bacon + Veg, 61
    Non-Starchy Roasted Vegetables, 123
    Pan-Roasted Cauliflower with Caper-Currant Relish + Yogurt-Tahini Sauce, 128
    Pan-Sautéed Baby Turnips with Turnip Green Pesto, 127
    Roasted Honeynut Squash, 133
    Span-ish Frittata with Spinach, 138
    Starchy Roasted Vegetables, 123
    Steak Knife Roasted Vegetables, 122–23
    Super Green Veg + Fruit Shake, 50
    Toasted Plantain Crumbs for, 37
    Wild Mushrooms with Ghee, Herbs + Sherry Vinegar, 134
vinaigrette. *See* Marlit's Vinaigrette; Three Dressings
vinegar, about, xviii

walnuts
    Carrot Birthday Cake, 217–18
    Chicory Chop Salad, 77
    Grain-Free Granola, 54
    House Pesto, 10
    Turnip Green Pesto, 127
watercress, Salad, Mandarin, Avocado +, 81
White Bean + Chorizo Stew, 99
Whole Garlic Prawns with Charred Lemon, 159
Whole Roasted Branzino, 151
Whole-Lemon Anchovy Dressing, 9, 77
Wild Blueberry Muffins, 58
Wild Fried Fish Tacos with Quick Pickled Slaw + Chipotle Aioli, 156–57
Wild Mushrooms with Ghee, Herbs + Sherry Vinegar, 134
wild tuna fish, about, xviii

yellow squash, Cacio e Pepe 2.0, 113
yogurt. *See* coconut yogurt
Yogurt-Tahini Sauce, 128
yuca. *See* cassava flour

Za'atar Toasted Pepitas, 34, 133
zucchini
    Crispy Brussels Sprouts with Fish Sauce Caramel, 124
    Turkey Zucchini Patties with Coconut Yogurt Tzatziki, 177

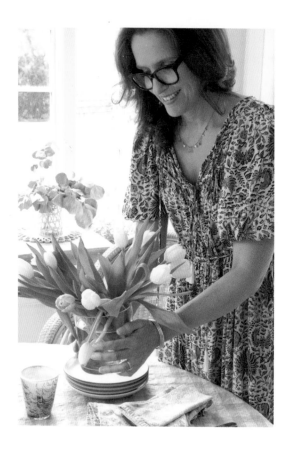

About the Author

Chay Wike grew up in New York City. Her parents and grandparents are from Cape Town, South Africa. From a young age she had the privilege of traveling overseas to visit family and was exposed to all kinds of cultures and eating styles. Her path to healing began after the birth of her second child, when she was diagnosed with multiple autoimmune conditions, digestive issues, and, eventually, Lyme disease. Following a string of doctor visits, confusion, and failed medication attempts, Chay decided to take matters into her own hands and reclaim her health naturally. She has since mostly recovered using the undeniable power of functional nutrition and lifestyle medicine. She attended cooking school in Los Angeles in 2009, created the food-focused wellness blog *The Kitchen Commune* in 2018, and became a certified integrative nutrition health coach in 2020. Today, Chay lives in the Pennsylvania countryside with her husband and their two teenage daughters.